# Comparative and Cross-cultural Health Research

## A practical guide

John Øvretveit

RADCLIFFE MEDICAL PRESS

Radcliffe Medical Press Ltd
18 Marcham Road, Abingdon, Oxon OX14 1AA, UK

British Library Cataloguing in Publication Data

A catalogue record for this book is available from the British Library.

ISBN 1 85775 274 0

Typeset by Advance Typesetting Ltd, Oxon
Printed and bound by Biddles Ltd, Guildford and King's Lynn

# Contents

# Foreword

Comparisons are double-edged. Badly done, or pursued in the wrong frame of mind, comparisons mislead and can easily demoralise. Done well and motivated by the intention to learn, not to blame, the act of comparison can be a potent asset to support improvement.

This book is helpful in formalising and categorising this wide range of methods for comparison, but it is equally helpful for the messages that it sends to readers about the psychology of comparison. Professor John Øvretveit knows the difference between comparisons that help and those that do not. One of the most prolific and thoughtful writers in health care management and health services research today, Professor Øvretveit has produced a stream of useful articles and monographs exploring the intersections among such fields as general management organisational psychology, research design and quality improvement. He is by nature and intellectual bent a builder of bridges. With a mature and respectful regard for the pressures and constraints that shape the world of today's health care leaders throughout the Western nations, Øvretveit has taken upon himself the complex task of analysing and presenting the powerful frameworks of evaluative and experimental science in such a way that 'real world' day-to-day leaders can grasp and, if they wish, apply those frameworks to their own work in the service of their organisations.

In this book, Professor Øvretveit carefully explains how the act of comparison can be designed and executed so that valid and useful knowledge emerges. He rightly includes options that range across the whole spectrum of design. At one extreme are the formal approaches of quasi-experimental design that would be familiar to technical university-based researchers. At the other extreme are far less quantitative, but sometimes even more informative observational methods that merge smoothly into the narrative comparisons that modern quality improvement jargon calls 'benchmarking'.

In health care today, especially, the very idea of making comparison too often carries with it an implicit (or explicit) sense of threat. In this mode, comparison is the entryway to such sequelae as reward, punishment, criticism, censure or even ridicule. To compare the performance of two hospitals, two surgeons or two health systems with this psychological set is to assume that one is better and one is worse; that one deserves praise and the other blame; even that one deserves to survive and the other to wither. This view is prevalent. In some sectors of Western medicine, it is even dominant. But it is terribly naïve in its failure to respect both human motives and the dynamics of human learning.

A more sophisticated and far more helpful view, that embraced by Professor Øvretveit, is that making comparisons and deeply understanding what one finds is a powerful way to learn. Good coaches coach by helping their players observe differences. If you want to learn chess, observe the differences in approach among the masters. Indeed, if there were no differences, no variation, then learning itself would become at best rote and mindless.

Judgements for the purpose of reward and punishment provoke fear. Comparison for the purpose of learning need not. It is the job of good teachers and good leaders to make comparisons safe and informative. In this endeavour, both teachers and leaders will do well to have a careful look at this book by Professor Øvretveit. It will show them how to use the force of comparison scientifically to increase the base of knowledge in the service of improvement.

Donald M Berwick
President
Institute for Healthcare Improvement
*August 1998*

# Preface

Making comparisons is instinctive, but the instinct can easily get us into trouble – we are too quick to make comparisons that are not justified and reach the wrong conclusions. Scientific methods help us to develop our abilities to make valid comparisons.

In my career as a health researcher, and in running educational programmes at the Nordic School of Public Health and University of Bergen, I noticed an increase in the amount of comparative health research being undertaken. More health practitioners and researchers were carrying out comparative health research. There was a rise in interest in cross-national and cross-cultural research. I found myself running more programmes for health service researchers and supervising more students carrying out such research. However, there were no texts that covered the range of subjects studied in health service research, or described the variety of social and natural science methods which were used. The origins of this book lie in the need for such a text.

If it was only to teach research, this book would not have been written. It was the increasing use made by managers and clinicians of comparative research in their everyday decisions that gave the stimulus for the book. Comparisons allow us to discover the causes of disease, whether a treatment is effective, if it is worth the cost, whether a service is performing badly and the value of a health reform or policy. Yet it is all too easy to misinterpret a comparative study or uncritically accept the conclusions of a poor study. Poor comparisons are worse than none. One of the aims of this book is to encourage decision-makers to make more use of comparative research, but to do so with a fuller awareness of the limitations of a particular study.

Another reason for writing this book, and perhaps the best reason for reading at least some of it, is that comparative health research is a fascinating and stimulating subject. I hope the book conveys some of my own and other's interest for the subject, and I hope it makes readers more cautious and critical about comparative studies. We need to deepen our understanding of differences and similarities between cultures and services and not to reinforce our prejudices. I hope too that it stimulates you to carry out your own study and to make more use of the research which has been done.

John Øvretveit
*August 1998*

# An introduction to comparative health research

*Travel and information technology are changing our world. More comparisons are being made and more comparative research is being undertaken. Yet comparative health research is more difficult than other types of research, both conceptually and practically. Without research skills it is easy to misinterpret the conclusions. The purpose of this book is to help you to make better use of comparative studies and to carry out better comparative research.*

## Introduction

The book is for health researchers and people working in health services who use or may make a comparative research study. We frequently make and use comparisons, and the ability to do so properly is becoming more important. This book describes concepts and methods for comparing health, treatments, organisations, health systems, policies, health reforms and interventions to health organisations. It proposes that we can improve our abilities to make valid and useful comparisons by learning methods and principles that are common to research into all these diverse subjects, and by taking a multidisciplinary perspective.

Making comparisons is instinctive. Discerning differences and similarities is a psychological ability that is 'built in' to us, possibly because it gave us evolutionary advantage as a species. It is an ability which helps us to make sense of and adapt to our world (Kelly, 1955). But is making comparisons also a way of producing scientific knowledge, and knowledge which enables us to improve health and the working of health services? The answer proposed by this book is yes – as long as the research is carried out with care and using specific methods.

Scientific methods allow us to extend and develop our inherited cognitive abilities to make better comparisons and to explain similarities and differences. One example is testing a health treatment by comparing its effect on one group of people who receive a treatment with another group who do not. Many methods and principles for comparative health research will be familiar to anyone with a research training. However, comparative research – and especially cross-cultural research – is more demanding of conceptual and practical research skills than many other types of research. Greater care is needed in sampling, in ensuring valid and reliable data collection, and in recognising and assessing confounders. There are also particular problems in carrying out comparative research if we are using a phenomenological or subjectivist approach to social research. All too often the research design is set up to confirm prejudices rather than to make new discoveries.

Comparative research is different to other research in ways that have not been sufficiently recognised in the literature. There are few texts that those interested in comparative health research can turn to for ideas and guidance, and none that apply to the range of subjects and disciplines within health research. This text aims to give an introduction to comparative health research for both researchers and users of research, such as managers, policy-makers and practitioners. Some of the ideas discussed will also be of help to those running comparative learning programmes, such as exchange visits and action learning courses for managers. The book considers how to maximise the learning from such programmes.

# Easier access to information and standardisation does not itself ensure good comparative research

Comparative research is a growing field, but is it of more value than other types of research? Are comparative learning visits worth the extra time and cost compared to other activities? The answer given by this book is a qualified 'yes' – sometimes, and under certain circumstances and for particular purposes. Invalid comparisons are common, both in research and in learning visits. The easier availability of information and cross-national databases is leading to more comparisons, but not necessarily better ones. In the past, comparative research and learning has been automatically viewed as a 'good thing' and is often subject to less rigorous criteria than other types of research and learning. There is too quick a tendency to assume that differences are due to differences in 'culture' – that catch-all concept often used to explain everything – rather than being due to differences in data collection.

This book takes the view that it is now incumbent on advocates to prove the value of comparative methods and to improve the quality of comparative studies. It starts with the 'null hypothesis' that all comparisons are invalid, and that comparative research is worse than useless because it diverts time and resources from other more useful and valid research. It is only by taking a more critical approach that we can develop this approach to research and learning.

## Improving comparative methodology and research through interdisciplinary co-operation

One way to improve comparative health research is through greater interdisciplinary co-operation. Other disciplines have often faced and solved the conceptual or practical problems that we face in a study we are doing – problems which we might not have even recognised. For example, epidemiologists have learnt from the methods used by Durkhiem in his 1897 study of the sociology of suicide. There is much that health researchers can learn from the debate in psychology about cross-cultural intelligence and personality testing, and from the methods and designs developed by psychologists: these ideas can be used directly to enhance the use of patient-testing instruments in comparative health research.

We can also learn from linguistics and anthropology about the problems and solutions in understanding cultural differences and in making valid comparisons about behaviour and attitudes between cultures. Organisational sociology and business administration have for some time wrestled with problems comparing organisations and in cross-cultural research, and have developed solutions that are not known in the health field. In a practical sense, management science can also help us with techniques to manage projects that involve research teams from different countries. Many comparative studies that go beyond description to explanation will usually need to draw on a variety of disciplines to understand the influences that might account for any similarities or differences found in the study.

The proposal, then, is that we can learn from other disciplines and that we need to improve both our abilities and our methods for using and carrying out comparative research.

## Why the growth of comparative research?

Information technology, the globalisation of markets and corporations, easier travel, greater cultural awareness and greater cultural uniformity are some of the often contradictory trends that are changing our world. On the one hand there is increasing globalisation and uniformity as a result of travel and communications. On the other there is increasing fragmentation and awareness of differences and diversity. These and other trends are affecting our health, our perceptions of wellbeing, our health systems and our expectations of health services.

Patients compare the treatments they receive with those they read about that are available elsewhere. The commerce in ideas has never been greater and more rapid: policy-makers may be more knowledgeable about the changes of policy and health system reforms taking place in a country on the other side of the world than the changes in a neighbouring region. With the speed of change, and greater insecurity, patients, policy-makers and managers turn to science for answers and certainty. If comparisons are to be made and if our services and treatments are to be compared to others, then should not these comparisons be scientific, or at least not misleading? With the changes that are occurring comes a perhaps naive belief that comparisons are one solution to the confusion and uncertainties of the modern world.

## Outline of this book

Before we discuss methods in the 'tool box' of comparative research, we first consider why we make and use comparisons in the health sector: which problems and questions can comparisons help us with? This is one of the questions considered in this introductory chapter, which also gives examples of the different types of subjects studied using a comparative approach. The chapter also gives examples of successful and unsuccessful comparative research, notes some of the problems and gives a way to represent and summarise a study in a diagram.

Chapter 2 divides comparative health research into eight categories. Starting with the category of 'comparisons of population health needs', it gives examples of studies within each category. We see from examples of comparisons of health treatments, systems, policies and other subjects that we can learn useful methods from disciplines and fields with which we may not be familiar. Chapter 3 shows how comparisons help us with two of the tasks of scientific research: to describe and explain. It describes the purposes of different types of study, including those that seek to find underlying similarities in phenomena that appear at first sight to be different ('genotypical' research). We also consider the empiricist, positivist and subjectivist research perspectives in comparative health research. We see that our research perspectives and values influence the type of questions we ask. The chapter also gives a simple but effective way of summarising and making sense of a comparative study – to draw a diagram of it.

One of the themes of the book is that we need to be clear about our questions and the purposes of the research in order to decide whether we need to use a comparative approach, and to choose the right methods. Chapter 4 develops this point and gives criteria for assessing a comparative study and guidance for planning a study. 'How do we make a valid comparison?' is a question addressed by describing six aspects of a research study, starting with how to define the research question and finishing with how to formulate valid conclusions.

Given the many subjects and purposes of comparative health research, we would expect many different types of research design. In fact most studies use one of eight types of design. Chapter 5 describes these designs, the strengths and weaknesses of each, and gives examples. An understanding of design is not just necessary for researchers. We see that, when first reading a comparative study, it helps to decide which type of design the study uses. This allows us quickly to make sense of the study and also to recognise its inherent limitations.

Data gathering is at the centre of most research, and comparative research is no exception. It is exceptional in the care and attention that needs to be paid by researchers to how the traditional methods of data gathering are used, if they are to make valid comparisons. Chapter 6 shows the extra precautions that need to be taken and the traps that lie in wait when using already-collected data and when using other methods for gathering data in comparative research, such as questionnaires and interviews.

Chapter 7 continues the practical discussion by considering some of the issues in planning and carrying out a comparative study. As with data gathering, the practical issues and logistics of comparative research are often more complicated than for other types of research, especially for cross-national studies with multiple research teams.

In the rest of this chapter we consider definitions of comparative- and cross-area health research. We look at some of the purposes of this type of research and note some of the subjects and questions that are studied through making comparisons between different areas, populations and institutions. We look at some of the drawbacks and difficulties, then present a model that allows us to analyse and represent any comparative research study. This model introduces some basic concepts which we will be using in the rest of the book: the concept of the 'whole object' (e.g. a population) and 'characteristics' of it (e.g. a disease) that are compared, and the 'context' or environment of the 'whole object' (e.g. the economic or cultural context).

# Definitions and purposes of comparative health research

*What is comparative health research? How does it differ from other types of research? What are the purposes and the subjects of such research?*

There is a whole family of activities that fall under the heading of 'comparative health research' (CHR). A broad definition is research that creates empirical or explanatory knowledge about health, health services or health systems, by making comparisons using scientific methods that are appropriate for the subject studied and for the purpose of the research. The aim of such research is to explore or explain the similarities and differences between comparable 'items' in different areas in order to improve health and the functioning of health services.

One common type is 'cross-area comparative health research' (CACHR). Examples include:

- a comparison of the incidence of influenza in an urban and a rural region of Denmark

- a comparison of hospital financing systems in Norway and Sweden

- a comparison of two methods that are used in primary care services for measuring health service quality.

The aim of this type of research is to discover whether an 'item' exists in different areas, to describe similarities and differences between items in different areas or to explain the item in relation to its context. The aim is to understand or explain the phenomenon and to inform the actions of practitioners, managers or health-policy-makers.

The 'items' compared in CHR and CACHR include 'entities' (e.g. organisations or health systems), 'events' or 'phenomena' (e.g. death, disease, health needs, some policies such as patients' rights) or processes over time (e.g. disease progression, interventions to organisations, health policies and reforms). The aims are to enable people to make better decisions than they would otherwise make, to sensitize people to issues they may not have considered, to broaden thinking and to contribute to empirical or explanatory scientific knowledge.

## Comparative learning

There is another activity that involves systematic comparisons and which can draw on methods used in comparative health research. Comparative learning is developing a person or group's knowledge, skills or attitudes by enabling them to understand and explain similarities and differences between health services, policies or health states and to draw conclusions for their own actions. Examples of comparative learning include:

- action learning visits, exchanges, networks and consultancy projects which involve comparisons and which are undertaken for the learner's development (Øvretveit, 1997b)

- 'best practices' programmes (e.g. the Australian 'Lighthouse model' hospital projects).

## Management technology transfer

Another subfield within comparative research is management technology transfer – a rapidly developing applied subdiscipline, which draws on the methods of evidence-based health care (Øvretveit, 1997c). This involves a set of methods to identify and transfer management methods and solutions which have been used successfully in one setting to another setting. An example is a set of systematic methods for seeking out and adapting solutions to a quality problem faced by a hospital, and for sensitising hospital quality project leaders to issues and problems they might face ('quality transfer technology'; QTT) (Øvretveit, 1997c).

This book concentrates on methods for making comparisons between 'items' in different nations, geographical areas or cultures. It does not consider comparisons of one item over time, such as a comparison of the state of health of a population in one area before and after an epidemic. These types of comparisons are already discussed in detail in existing texts on health services research and evaluation (e.g. Holland, 1983; St Leger *et al.*, 1992; Øvretveit, 1998).

## Purpose and aims of comparative health research

The above definitions give a sense of how comparative health research differs from other types of activity. We can deepen and extend this introduction by noting some of the purposes of comparative research studies. These are to explore, interpret or explain the similarities and differences between comparable items or phenomena in different areas, in order to improve health and the functioning of health services. The aim is one or more of the following:

- to discover whether an event, phenomena or entity that occurs in one place also occurs in another (e.g. do residents of Iceland and Greenland suffer from 'seasonal affective disorder' as do residents of northern Norway? Do general practitioners hold budgets to purchase health care in Sweden as well as in the UK?)

- to discover 'significant' similarities or differences between comparable 'items' in different areas (e.g. are arrangements for 'decentralised budgets' the same in different hospitals or health systems?)

- to measure the size differences or gather data about the meaning of the 'items' or phenomena in different areas (e.g. are 'community hospitals' the same size in different Nordic countries? How do recent immigrants in Sweden react to the diagnosis of breast cancer compared to Swedish-born residents?)

- to understand, interpret or explain the similarities or differences between items in different places (e.g. why are there differences in the way hospitals implement a particular law or regulation?)

- to contribute to decisions about actions to improve health or the functioning of health services (e.g. by comparing the different success of the same training programme in different places we can improve the training programme with guidelines for how to implement it differently in different organisations)

- to contribute to the adoption of improved practices or procedures by comparing a new more effective procedure to one customarily used elsewhere, or by comparing how commonly a practice is used in different areas and the reasons for the difference.

# Examples and subjects

*Which types of questions can comparative research help us with?*

*What are the subjects of comparative research studies?*

To give a flavour of the type of research we will be considering, we list here some general questions that have been addressed and some example studies. In Chapter 4 we will look at how important it is to define a clear question or testable hypothesis if we are to carry out useful comparative research. Defining the question also helps us to check whether making a comparison is in fact the best way of producing the required knowledge.

# Some questions addressed by comparative health research studies

- Are there significant differences in mortality and morbidity in Europe, and if so, why?

- Do Norwegians sleep better than Russians in the northern Svalbard region?

- For comparable areas of Sweden and England, why are there twice as many doctors and nurses per head of population in the Swedish area and twice as much spent on health care, and is the Swedish people's health better as a result?

- Are Swedish people more satisfied with their health service than Danish and British people?

- Are there differences in rates of psychiatric morbidity in different Nordic countries, differences in rates of presentation of such illnesses in primary care and differences in rates of diagnosis by GPs?

- How useful are international and area comparisons of medical care utilisation such as surgery rates?

- Why are there such large differences in the proportion of home to hospital births in Sweden and Denmark, and what can we learn from comparing the changes in place of birth since the 1890s and the reason for these changes?

- Are there differences in the costs of treatments provided by comparable private and public hospitals, in the quality of care and, if so, why are there these differences?

- What are the different health reforms that European countries have introduced in the last five years and what have been the results?

- How have Norway and Finland tried to reduce regional inequities in health and in access to health care?

- What can we learn from comparing the way in which knowledge about sudden infant death syndrome was diffused in different countries?

- What are current best practices in management and clinical practice and how might managers and clinicians identify these and apply them to their own setting?

**Table 1.1**: Examples of comparative research studies to illustrate the range of subjects and methods

| Comparison of | Summary | Reference |
|---|---|---|
| Health needs (Mental health needs and demands in areas within five Nordic countries) | Study of hidden psychiatric morbidity and prevalence of psychiatric illness in 1281 patients consulting GPs in a Nordic multicentre study | Fink *et al.* (1995) |
| Mortality (Cardiovascular mortality) | Comparison of cardiovascular mortality and discussion of differences and possible causes | Rosen & Thelle (1996) |
| Health differences | Uses WHO and European Union databases to compare health in 12 European countries, and considers their differences in terms of a model of determinants of health. Short discussion of data limitations and the need for European standardisation | Schaapveld *et al.* (1995) |
| Health-related behaviour (Suicide) | Comparison within Sweden of the effect on suicide rates of immigration, ethnicity, age, sex and marital status, using central 'Cause of Death Register' and 1985 Swedish census | Johansson *et al.* (1997) |

**Table 1.1**: Continued

| Comparison of | Summary | Reference |
|---|---|---|
| Treatments (Variations in surgical rates) | Comparison of rates for common surgical procedures in New England, England and Norway, using hospital data reported to regional centres, standardised for age and sex | McPherson et al. (1982) |
| Service performance (Activity and outputs) | A comparison of Scottish hospitals for 1991 using data describing inpatient or day-case discharges from gynaecological units as well as data from Scottish Morbidity Records Form 1. The study shows the importance when making comparisons between outcomes of taking into account characteristics of patients, diagnostic case mix and the social circumstances of the area | Leyland & Boddy (1997) |
| Interventions to health services | Six hospital quality programmes compared | Øvretveit & Aslaksen (1998) |
| Health reforms | Comparison of health reforms in the OECD countries | Hurst (1992) |
| Health policies (To reduce inequalities in health and accessibility) | Comparison of the implementation of policy to decrease regional differences in health status and accessibility to health services. Compares data on inequalities from existing sources, and notes the limitations of these sources | Samela (1993) |
| Other types of comparisons (Comparability of different economic evaluations undertaken in different countries) | The same economic evaluation of a drug was undertaken in four countries using the same methods. This study considers whether a standard method could be agreed in different countries to ensure comparability of findings and to compare differences in costs and benefits in different countries | Drummond et al. (1992) |

## Categories of comparative health research

The comparisons we consider in this book are those that enable us to improve health and health services. We can see from the examples that the subjects of comparative health research studies are many and various. A study may take as the subject for comparison the same disease in different populations, or it may compare organisations, training programmes, health policies and health service reforms, to name just a few. The subjects of comparative research can be:

- health states, behaviour, attitudes and other characteristics of individuals or populations

- health treatments

- health services (which include methods of assessment and one or more treatments carried out for a defined group of patients)

- health organisations or subunits (e.g. teams, departments, hospitals, primary health care units, purchasing or financing organisations, regulatory or inspection agencies, patient associations and professional associations)

- health systems (local, regional or national)

- health policies, health care policies or health reforms

- interventions to health organisations (e.g. training programmes, changes to structure or quality of programmes).

The above list of subjects is a way of categorising comparative health research studies in terms of the type of subject that is compared. Chapter 2 defines each category and gives examples of studies; a longer list is given in Appendix 4. Chapter 3 considers the different research paradigms used to study these subjects.

Similar research methods are used to study subjects in each category, and these methods are often different to those used for studying subjects in another category. For example, studies that compare health states of different populations use similar methods, but these methods are different to those used in studies to compare health reforms. Surely the differences between these subjects mean that the strategies for research into each have little in common? What value is there in concentrating on methods for comparison when the way in which these methods are applied in different types of research is so great?

This book proposes that there are many methods and concepts for making comparisons that are common across all these subjects. There is much to be learnt about methods of comparison from disciplines with which we are not familiar. It suggests that a 'transdiscipline' of comparative health research is emerging, which will increasingly contribute to health services practice, management and policy-making.

There is, however, an alternative view which holds that improvements in comparative methods are best pursued within each discipline; that the methods and subjects are so different that there is little that can be learnt from the approaches to comparison used in other disciplines. At this point we need to note the different research perspectives in health services research because this has a bearing on whether there is value in looking at methods for comparison accross such a diverse field. We will return to the more tangible question of 'why make comparisons?'

## Different approaches to research and types of subjects

There are different philosophical assumptions about the nature of the subject studied which underlie different approaches to comparative research. In health research we can conceptualise our subject as a physical object, as a human subject or as a collective social object or process.

If we think of a person as a physical object, we concentrate on biochemical, physiological and physical processes which operate according to general laws and can be understood in terms of causation. The 'natural science' approach has a long history in health research, and the assumptions have been characterised as 'empiricist' or 'positivist' – assumptions about the nature of 'facts' and about how empirical and explanatory knowledge of the 'real world' can be produced. Empiricism holds that 'facts speak for themselves' and that the real world can be apprehended directly. Positivism holds that we need pre-observational concepts to help us gather data directly from the real world. Science should gather data to refute hypotheses derived from theory and in this way build up knowledge of increasing certainty. This perspective is most often applied to investigating diseases and influences on health at the individual and population level, and where a person or population can be regarded as a physical object subject to causal mechanisms.

We can also think of a person as a conscious subject, in the sense of being able to give meaning and value to their experiences and to events in the world. The 'subjectivist' approach holds that, in many areas of existence, people can choose how they act and are not determined by causal influences.

This approach to health research argues that, to explain both individual acts and many social phenomena, we have to understand how people interpret events. We have to collect data about subjective meanings in order to construct explanations for both individual and collective actions.

We also need to understand subjective meanings and actions in terms of a particular context and culture which makes them intelligible; acts and understandings are rule-governed, even though we create and recreate the rules in our actions. Comparative research thus involves considering the contexts of individual and social actions in order to understand any differences and similarities in how people act and interpret the world. Indeed, there are those working within this perspective who argue that comparison is invalid and behaviour and rules are unique to a particular culture and time. The methods used to understand the context and people's acts and ideas are different to those used in natural sciences to study physical objects. The way we collect data and construct explanations is different to that used in the natural sciences.

The point of raising these issues here is to note that there are different perspectives in health services research, and the research perspective affects both how one carries out and how one understands a comparative study. The approach taken by this book is not to argue for or against a particular perspective, but to highlight the issues. Each approach can bring insights. For example, a disease process in an individual can be understood in terms of the subjective meanings given to the disease by the person, which in turn is influenced by the culture of which they are part. These meanings may even affect the course of the disease, but most diseases also progress according to predictable processes which can be illuminated by taking a natural-science perspective. A cross-cultural study can help to disentangle the cultural and biological determinants of a particular disease process.

Generally, the approach taken in this book could be called a 'dualist' or mixed approach: that individuals and social entities are influenced by factors about which they may not be aware, and which may be understood as having a 'causal effect' on them which show law-like regularities. But individuals and social groups are also able to understand some of these influences and to choose not to be determined by some or to accommodate others and give meaning to these influences.

There has been considerable debate about which approach is 'best' for studying social phenomena and social entities such as hospitals, health policies and health systems. Should these subjects be studied using natural-science methods and should we seek to explain events in terms of laws and causation? Or should these subjects be studied using methods to discover the subjective perceptions and values of individuals and groups, and events explained in terms of how people give meaning to events?

We will return to these questions in Chapter 4. The main points at this stage are: there are many different subjects studied in health services research; and there are at least two ways of conceptualising many of the subjects of comparative research – from an objectivist or subjectivist perspective, each perspective having different methods and aims. Finally, the research approach taken depends on the purpose and questions of the research.

# Why compare?

*Why is more comparative research being undertaken, and what are the benefits of this type of research?*

Travel and information systems are changing our world and making it both easier and more necessary to understand cultural differences. There is an increasing practical need for knowledge from cross-national and cross-cultural health research. Clinicians are treating more people from different countries and different ethnic groups. Planners and policy-makers need to understand the different rates of disease in different populations and how to ensure accessibility to services for different ethnic groups, as well as other sources of regional and ethnic inequality. Health managers can improve their services by sensitively adapting ideas that have worked elsewhere, and by avoiding other's mistakes. They too need to understand cultural differences to serve patients and manage employees from different nations and ethnic groups.

Comparative health research has a part to play in relieving suffering: by using systematic comparison to create scientific knowledge about causes of ill health and about effective methods for care, cure and health promotion. It also has a role in building relations between nations and different communities, by creating knowledge that helps people understand their similarities and differences to other peoples. It builds bridges in a small way in comparative learning programmes and in researcher collaboration in cross-area research projects.

However, the time and money invested in a comparative research study needs to be justified: such studies often consume more resources than other types of research and a comparative study might not be necessary to answer the research question or give any added value. Some more specific reasons for undertaking comparative research include:

- generating empirical scientific knowledge about similarities and differences which can form the basis for explanatory knowledge of causes or for understanding influences

- meta-analysis: comparing the results of studies to build a broader or deeper knowledge of a subject

- generating knowledge for clinicians about diseases in different ethnic groups and populations; the prevalence, incidence and cultural influences in presentation and treatment (e.g. cross-cultural psychiatry)

- assisting changes to practice by showing that other practitioners or services use different methods and get better results, and by stimulating a questioning attitude

- contributing to open-mindedness for change by showing that familiar practices and roles are not the only way

- discovering differences in costs or quality of care between comparable hospitals, services and patient conditions to stimulate managers to investigate the reasons for the differences

- improving management and organisation by discovering and describing more efficient or effective practices and organisation elsewhere, and by showing the possible scope for improvement

- increasing managers' understanding of how to manage employees from different ethnic groups and how to maximise creativity from diversity in the workforce

- learning from and avoiding mistakes which others have made elsewhere, and replicating their successes

- contribute to policy formulation by comparing policies in other countries and making use of natural experiments elsewhere, hence avoiding the political problems of high visibility with a pilot testing within one country

- development of research methods and of researchers; comparative research often involves interdisciplinary and multidisciplinary cooperation which can contribute to new research methods and can also help to train researchers from countries which have few researchers or research training programmes. Learning how to carry out comparative research also sensitises researchers to problems in conventional research which they may not have been aware of, and shows in a clear form common issues encountered in other types of research.

# Benefits of and examples of successful comparative health research

One indication of the perceived value of comparisons is the resources invested by international organisations in collecting, publishing and analysing comparative data. Extensive and detailed comparative health and health-related data are collected and published, as well as analyses of these data, by the Nordic Council (e.g. NOMESCO, 1996; NCM, 1995), the European Commission (CEC, 1988; Eurostat, 1992), the Organisation for Economic Cooperation and Development (OECD, 1990, 1993a,b, 1994; Hurst, 1992), the World Bank (WB, 1993) and the World Health Organisation (1992, 1997). There are also many regularly published within-nation comparisons of health and of health service performance (e.g. the UK NHS performance indicators and 'hospital league tables'). The large amount of data now readily available, and the effort being put into standardisation and improving these data, indicates that these organisations and their sponsors believe in the value of comparisons for policy-making and other purposes.

Using these databases, and also by collecting their own data, a number of researchers have carried out successful comparative research which has had a real practical impact. Some examples include:

- International comparison of disease: a comparison of the prevalence of non-insulin-dependent diabetes found large differences (e.g. Indonesia 1.7%, American Pima Indians 25.5%). This contributed to further studies to find causes related to country or ethnic background and to diabetic services planning for different populations (WHO, 1994b, 1995).

- International and local comparisons of variation in surgical operation rates contributed to lowering of inappropriate surgery in areas where the 'high' rates were publicised (Domenighetti *et al.*, 1988).

- Comparison of health, socioeconomic and other factors in different areas led to the creation of health-related 'deprivation indices' for more equitable resource allocation in the UK (Jarman, 1983).

- Comparison of the experiences of different hospitals with different quality systems led to a change of emphasis from ISO 9000 systems towards other quality improvement methods (Joss & Kogan, 1995; Øvretveit, 1994b).

- Comparison of the adoption of health policies and practices for preventing sudden infant death in different countries led to new, more effective approaches being adopted.

- Comparison of different methods for rationing and prioritising has contributed to national and international debate, improvements to methods and fairer systems (Honingsbaum *et al.*, 1996).

## Examples of less successful comparative health research

However, there are also examples of unsuccessful and misleading research, and perhaps more of it than other types of research because the problems of comparison are not as well understood or obvious. Some examples of less successful comparisons include:

- Poor comparison of a health-related behaviour in a 14-country study. The reader is invited to imagine the reliability of the data produced by each of the 14 sets of researchers and busy psychiatrists when following this operational definition:

  *Parasuicide is defined in the study as an act with non-fatal outcome, in which an individual deliberately initiates a non-habitual behaviour that, without intervention from others, will cause self-harm, or deliberately ingests a substance in excess of the prescribed or generally recognised therapeutic dosage, and which is aimed at realising changes which she desired via the actual or expected physical consequences.*

- Comparison of national health expenditure which did not recognise changes in classification. Services for older people were removed from health expenditure calculations in Sweden in 1992 following the Adel reforms which transferred responsibilities from counties to communes, yet some international comparisons did not take this into account.

- Comparison of outcomes of cancer treatments at different centres. The subjects were not randomly allocated and those for the 'alternative cancer treatment' had a longer experience of illness.

- Comparison of internal market reforms without considering context. The relative success of the UK NHS market reforms were compared with those for the Nordic countries without discussion of the UK context. This context included the previous 10 years of health management development, the centralised direction with no local democracy and the strength of traditional NHS values and culture, all of which moderated the managed competition in the system that was introduced.

# Problems

*What are some of the problems and difficulties in using and making comparisons?*

The benefits and advantages of comparative research are not achieved without a cost. It is difficult and expensive to carry out such research, and some comparative studies do not take sufficient precautions to ensure that the comparisons and explanations are valid. After reviewing a number of cross-national studies of health systems Elling (1994) commented that:

*Data sources are highly problematic in this field, depending as they do on official government reports which often serve 'image' purposes more than the truth. I have more faith in and recommend in-depth historical case studies, in which data can be contextually assessed, rather than cross-sectional correlation studies and multination surveys.* (Elling, 1994)

To date, many comparative studies using these data have been 'suggestive' and 'interesting', rather than conclusive. In relation to economic comparisons, an editorial in *Social Sciences and Medicine* (1993, **38**(1), vii) asked, 'is there any evidence of the performance of current health care systems in terms of efficiency and equity?', and answered:

*Despite three decades of health economics, there is still little evidence to suggest which model is to be preferred in what circumstances and there are indeed few rigorous comparative studies of health care. This is not surprising as international health care data are notoriously unreliable and difficult to interpret.*

The problems are not confined to economic comparisons. In part, the gap between the potential and the achievements may be because of limitations in existing data comparability (OECD, 1990), but there are questions as to how useful even well-standardised and reliable data are for some purposes of comparison. Indeed, the increasing availability of these data without the corresponding skills to use them brings its own problems. These problems are not necessarily resolved when researchers gather their own data directly. We return to these questions in Chapters 4 and 6.

Problems are usually greater in comparisons of such subjects as health systems, reforms, policies and interventions to organisations. Problems include the ambiguity and general terms in which some policies and reforms are described, difficulties in finding out when a policy was actually implemented, the extent of the implementation (breadth and depth), the phasing of a reform (e.g. UK fundholding), whether the plans for the policy and consultations themselves produced changes, reforms being in fact multiple changes (e.g. UK 1991 NHS reforms) and other changes taking place at the same time making it difficult to attribute possible effects and to make comparisons. When introducing their comparison of health care reforms in six countries, Ham *et al.* (1990) warn that, 'comparative analysis is more helpful in illustrating the problems that are common to different systems and the variations in policy responses than in suggesting solutions that can be transplanted between systems'.

The results of a comparative research study can be misleading for 'non-researcher users' or those not familiar with the methods. There are both methodological and practical problems.

## Threats to valid comparisons

Threats to valid comparisons and to valid explanations for similarities and differences come from:

- cultural or national differences affecting whether a health state is considered a disease or not; criteria for disease depend on definitions of normality and abnormality which differ between countries. International classifications do not fully overcome these problems

- poor selection of the items which are compared (e.g. populations or organisations not comparable)

- the same concept being operationalised differently in different countries (e.g. suicide), or subjects in different areas understanding different things by the same concept or word even when carefully translated

- unreliable data-gathering methods and difficulties standardising the data-gathering methods between areas (e.g. *see* Rosen, 1987)

- problems in controlling for confounding variables or failure to recognise context differences which affect or explain the phenomena in different places.

## Practical problems

Organising and managing a project with researchers or data-gathering from different areas is more difficult and takes longer than many other types of research, especially if there are linguistic differences. There are also practical problems in securing finance and resources for comparative research. Some institutions that carry out research give a lower priority to comparative research because it is not viewed as benefiting the host country or the institution. There is sometimes the opposite problem: that comparative research is encouraged without careful and knowledgeable assessment of the methods and prospects for success – the enthusiasm exceeds experience with, and critical assessment of, this type of research.

# What do we compare? Concepts and a model of a comparative study

*We do not compare the entities as such, but characteristics or concepts of entities.*

In this penultimate section of the chapter we introduce some concepts for describing and analysing a comparative research study. First we look at the different types of 'things' which are compared, and then at a way to represent and summarise a study by drawing a diagram of the design it uses.

## The nature of the subjects of comparative research

We saw from the earlier examples that comparative health research is a field that covers many different subjects. Some of these subjects can be described as 'entities' and some as 'characteristics', 'events', 'phenomena' or 'processes'. Up to now we have used the general term 'item' for the 'thing' that is compared. However, it is helpful to make a distinction between a 'whole object' and a 'characteristic' or dimension of a whole object (*see* Box 1.1).

---

**Box 1.1: Distinction between 'whole objects' and characteristics of 'whole objects'**

| *Whole object examples* | *Characteristic examples* |
|---|---|
| A person | Health needs, disease, perception of health |
| Population | Death rates, disease rates |
| Hospital | Size, management structure, performance |
| Health system | Ownership of health services, financing |
| Health policy | Purpose of the policy, who it is intended for |
| Health policy implementation process | Timescale, financing, decision-makers |

---

Some 'whole objects' can be described as 'entities', for example human populations or organisations. Some 'whole objects' are actually better described as processes, such as policy implementation process; 'object' is not the best term for a sequence of activities over time. Comparative research does not compare the entities as such, but compares characteristics or concepts of entities – one or more aspects of the entities such as a disease in a population or the management structure of a hospital. We consider later some of the problems of abstracting a characteristic from its context to make a comparison, especially if we are taking a systems perspective.

This point is easier to see in research that defines the concepts before data-gathering, as in experimental or epidemiological research; a concept or variable is defined, which is the dimension on which the entities are compared. This is less obvious in exploratory research, where entities are compared in order to discover ways in which the entities are similar and different. In this type of research, the researchers start with a loose definition of the entity  they will investigate. They build up concepts at one site as well as interacting with other researchers at other sites to build up concepts through comparisons ('comparative grounded theory' and 'comparative inductive research'). The point is that researchers do not compare reality as such, but gather data about concepts of an aspect of reality.

We return to these issues in Chapter 4, but here we need to note that the subject of comparison is termed 'item', regardless of whether the item is a whole object or a characteristic of it. 'Item' is thus the very general term used to refer to the 'thing' that is compared, be it disease, population, organisation, training programme, financing method, etc.

## Is the comparison context-independent?

In the following we introduce a model for representing a comparative research study (Figure 1.1). The purpose of Figure 1.1 is to draw attention to the difference between two comparative research studies. In the first, the context of the item is, for the purposes of the research, the same. In the second, the context of each item is different. When we are making comparisons between items in the same area the 'conceptual problems' are usually less than if we are making cross-national comparisons where the context becomes more important. However, we must always be aware of the possibility of invalid conceptual comparisons even within one area.

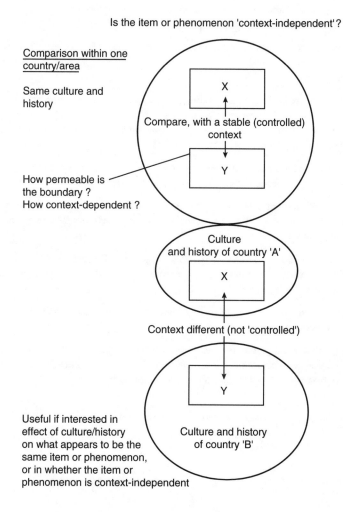

Is the item or phenomenon 'context-independent'?

Comparison within one
country/area

Same culture and
history

X

Compare, with a stable (controlled)
context

Y

How permeable is
the boundary ?
How context-dependent ?

Culture
and history of country 'A'

X

Context different (not 'controlled')

Y

Useful if interested in
effect of culture/history
on what appears to be the
same item or phenomenon,
or in whether the item or
phenomenon is context-independent

Culture and history
of country 'B'

**Figure 1.1** Two studies, with different contexts for the item

We will return to some of the issues raised by this diagram and the concepts of whole object and context in Chapter 4. We finish this chapter by summarising some of the terms used to describe comparative research studies.

---

**Box 1.2: Definitions**

*The 'whole object' or 'entity' which is compared*: two or more individuals, two or more populations, or organisations, systems, policies, or interventions to organisation.

*Characteristic*: a concept, dimension or variable which describes an aspect of the whole object which is compared – death, disease, levels of management, financing method, etc.

*Item*: a general term for that which is compared. The item may be a characteristic, or it may be a process. The item compared may also be a whole object or an entity, as for example in an exploratory study to discover any similarities and differences in an entity found in two or more places.

*Process comparison*: a comparison of changes over time in two or more entities, or a comparison of a sequence of activities carried out by or to an entity.

*Context*: the 'environment' surrounding the whole object, which is usually different in different areas, and which is conceptualised in terms of different factors or characteristics of context.

*Culture*: the combination of laws, customs, rules, language and ideas shared by a group of people and through which individuals express, understand and give meaning to their own and others' experiences.

*Data-gathering method*: a method used to gather data about an item, and to gather data about the context of the item.

*Boundary*: (a) that which separates the whole object from its context, and allows differentiation of the whole object and definition of it; (b) a term used to describe how the context is mediated to the item (e.g. causes operate on the whole object through a boundary).

*Design*: the overall research design, including sampling and how the items are compared.

---

## Summary – types of comparative health research

Comparative research studies can be described and categorised in terms of:

- the subject of study (termed here the 'whole object' and characteristics of it which are compared, such as health states, services, organisations, policies, etc.)

- the research approach (descriptive, explanatory, genotypical, phenotypical, experimental deductive, inductive theory/concept building; *see* Chapter 3)

- the design (Chapter 5)

- the way the research conceptualises the items compared (item boundaries fuzzy or clearly defined, item stable or changing, item interacts with context or relatively independent)

- disciplinary basis (policy comparison, economic, sociological, anthropological, epidemiological, etc.).

## Conclusions

- Comparative health research (CHR) is defined as research that creates empirical or explanatory knowledge about health, health services or health systems, by making comparisons using scientific methods that are appropriate for the subject studied and for the purpose of the research.

- The purpose of such research is to explore or explain the similarities and differences between comparable items or phenomena in different areas, in order to understand and improve health and the functioning of health services.

- Because the aim of CHR is to understand and improve health and health services, the subjects of CHR are many and varied, as are the research designs and data-gathering methods.

- The subjects of CHR studies include disease, health, behaviour, attitudes, treatments, services, interventions to health organisations, health systems, and health and health care policies. Although these subjects are very different in their nature, there are some principles and methods which apply to comparisons for all these subjects.

- CHR studies are carried out from different 'disciplinary bases', drawing on and contributing to theory or methods used in sociology, medical research, epidemiology, anthropology, management science, political science and policy studies. Some CHR studies are multidisciplinary in theory, method and researcher involvement, especially those that pay detailed attention to the context of the items compared.

- While there is diversity, there is also a distinct set of methods, theories and body of knowledge emerging – a 'transdiscipline' of comparative research. Improvements are needed and can be made by researchers learning from the methods and solutions to problems developed by researchers in other disciplines, and by more transdisciplinary comparative research.

- The problems in carrying out comparative research are similar to problems in most types of health research, but more acute. CHR provides a good introduction and learning examples for health researcher training.

- Rather than automatically assuming cross-national comparative research is of value, there is need to justify the extra expense. Such research can be improved by better designs and data-gathering methods and methodology, better project management, closer links with users of the research and by a more careful assessment of research proposals (*see* Chapter 4).

# 2

# Examples of comparative health research

## Introduction

This chapter divides comparative health research studies into eight categories and gives examples of studies within each category. The purposes of the chapter are threefold: to give an idea of the range of subjects and methods, to show what we can learn from comparative studies carried out by other disciplines into subjects with which we may not be familiar, and to highlight some of the strengths and weaknesses of comparative health research.

We consider comparisons of: population health needs, health states and behaviour, treatments, health services and organisations, interventions to health organisations, health systems, health reforms and both health policies and health care policies.

Each section follows a broadly similar format: a definition of the category of research, a note of the purpose of some studies within the category and an example. Each section also notes methodological issues and the lessons we can learn about making comparisons from studies within each category. Some of these are general lessons which apply to all types of comparative research; one of the themes of the book is that by looking beyond their own discipline, comparative researchers can often find methods and solutions developed in other fields that can be applied in their own. By considering these many types of research in one chapter we can see some of the potential for cross-disciplinary fertilisation and interdisciplinary working.

# Comparisons of population health needs

## Category definition

This category of research includes studies that compare the health needs of different populations. It includes within- and cross-country comparisons of the health needs of populations resident in different geographical areas, of different ethnic groups and of different age and sex groups.

## Purposes of comparative needs research

The purposes of comparative health needs research is to contribute to health planning and to decisions about purchasing, resource allocation and health policy, as well as to knowledge about inequities in health. This category overlaps with the next category of studies, which compares health states and health behaviour. However, the distinction between studies of health needs and studies of health is a necessary one. This is because financing and other agencies are increasingly carrying out health needs assessments for planning and resource allocation purposes, and a growing number of methods and concepts have been developed specifically for assessing and comparing health needs which are different to the more traditional methods for studying health and disease. Studies within this category sometimes use socioeconomic variables as indicators of health need because such indicators have been found to be associated with need for and demand for health care (Jarman, 1983; Townsend et al., 1988; Frohlich & Mustard, 1996).

Examples are studies using 'rapid appraisal' or 'rapid needs assessment' both in developed countries (Ong et al., 1991; Ong, 1993) and developing countries (Vlassoff & Tanner, 1992), as well as 'community diagnosis' (Rosen, 1987). The former combine epidemiological, demographic and socioeconomic data, as well as health-provider assessments and those of community and church groups. An example of a survey approach is that of Hopton and Dlugolecka (1995). This study surveyed patients registered with five Scottish general medical practices ($n = 3478$) to gather data about patients' reported health problems and other data. The study compared the different amounts and types of needs and demands of the patients registered with the different practices.

## Comparison of needs – an example study

Another example is a Nordic multicentre study of psychiatric morbidity in primary care. The study used different data-gathering methods to describe hidden psychiatric morbidity and the prevalence of psychiatric illness in 1281 patients consulting GPs in the different sites chosen for the study (Fink *et al.*, 1995; Munk-Jørgensen *et al.*, 1997). National differences in morbidity were found, but methodological problems meant that these could not be considered significant. Differences in GPs' abilities to recognise morbidity were significant, especially their ability to distinguish psychotic from non-psychotic illnesses.

There are lessons for other comparative health research from this study. These include the problems encountered, even in a carefully planned study, in ensuring that the same categories were used for recording data in each country, and how to define health needs (Bradshaw, 1972). The problems of valid comparison and cultural context are greater in comparative mental health research than in many other fields, and the concepts and methods developed can be used in other types of comparative research. In relation to the issue of how to define health needs, Bowling (1992, 1995) gives an overview of different methods that can be used in planning comparative needs assessment studies.

# Comparisons of health states and of health-related behaviour and attitudes

## Category definition

'Health state' in this book is a general term covering death (mortality), disease (morbidity), illness (subjective perception of 'unwellness'), quality of life, functional ability and disability. This category also includes comparisons of 'health-related behaviour', which is behaviour thought to affect health states, such as smoking, drinking alcohol, exercise and eating 'unhealthy food', and includes suicide. It also covers 'health-related attitude' comparisons, for example those which hypothesise that differences in health are associated with or due to differences in certain attitudes.

# Purposes of comparative research with this category

This is a category that encompasses a large and varied number of research studies, whose purposes can be summarised as describing and explaining differences and similarities in health in order to contribute to scientific knowledge and practical action.

Why would we want to compare the health states of individuals or populations within and between nations? One answer is that if we compare groups in different areas, which are the same in all respects apart from the fact that one group has a disease and the other group(s) do not, we may be able to discover something in people's life history or environment which might have caused the disease. If we compare two similar groups that both have the disease, we might be able to find that both have been exposed to the same events or environmental influences. Both of these reasons for comparing health states depend on having a hypothesis which we then test by one type of comparative design ('case comparative research', discussed in Chapter 5). Another reason for comparing health states is to find out if differences in health might be due to differences in health services or in access to health services.

There are many examples of descriptive databases that give comparisons of national mortality and morbidity data by different categories (Eurostat, 1992; WHO, 1992; OECD, 1993; NCM, 1995; NOMESCO, 1996). Examples of comparative studies that seek to go beyond description include a comparison of avoidable mortality in Eastern Europe (Boys *et al.*, 1991), an overview study of cardiovascular mortality in Nordic countries (Rosen & Thelle, 1996) and a comparative study of cancer mortality in central Europe (Evstifeeva *et al.*, 1997).

An example of a descriptive study that brings together a number of measures in a composite 'health expectancy indicator' is that of Boshuizen *et al.* (1994). This estimates and compares the number of years an average person can expect to live in good health during his or her lifetime in different European countries. There are also many comparative studies of health-related behaviour (e.g. alcohol consumption, WHO, 1992; tobacco consumption, World Bank, 1993) and health-related attitudes. There are fewer large-scale international comparisons of subjective perception or 'self-reports' of health (Schaapveld *et al.*, 1995). An interesting study of a health-related behaviour used data from the 1985 Swedish census and cause of death register to compare suicide rates of different immigrants and ethnic groups (Johansson *et al.*, 1997). One of the largest international comparative health studies of school-age children considered health attitudes in 19 European countries and Canada and Greenland (WHO, 1996a).

# Examples of comparative research studies within this category

The study by Schaapveld *et al.* (1995) is an ambitious one which goes beyond comparing descriptions of health in European countries (mortality, life expectancy, perceived health). It used a model of determinants of health to explain differences in health between 12 European countries. The model distinguishes five groups of determinants: hereditary, exogenous factors, socioeconomic and psychosocial factors, lifestyle and health care. The study used the WHO and European Union databases to compare health in European countries and discusses some of the limitations of these data. There are lessons for other comparisons from their discussion of the use of these databases and also from their attempt to explain the differences.

Both the potential of cross-national research and the methodological issues are well demonstrated in a set of studies into 11 900 men of Japanese ancestry (Marmot & Syme, 1976). The study aimed to compare coronary heart disease (CHD) in Japanese men in Japan, Hawaii and California, and relate these rates to risk factors. The study showed that 'the culture in which the individual is raised affects his likelihood of manifesting coronary heart disease in adult life', and that the relationship of culture of upbringing to CHD was independent of risk factors. The study found that the closer people adhered to traditional values, the lower their likelihood of CHD, and speculated as to whether a stable society and close support protected against the stress which could lead to CHD.

# Treatment comparisons

## Category definition

'Treatment' here refers to pharmaceutical and surgical interventions, as well as specific caring, rehabilitation and palliative practices, and specific diagnostic and assessment procedures. It does not refer to combinations of practices organised into what is termed below 'a service', although the distinction between 'treatment' and 'service' is not clear-cut.

This category of research includes many treatment evaluations involving comparisons between an 'experimental' and a 'control' group (e.g. those receiving placebo or conventional treatment) and all economic treatment evaluations. It also covers studies that compare variations in treatment and in pharmaceutical prescription rates between areas, as well as meta-evaluations which compare research evaluations of the same treatment in different countries.

## Purposes of comparative research with this category

The purposes of most research that compares a treatment with conventional treatment (or none at all) are to test hypotheses about effectiveness, or to calculate cost-effectiveness or cost utility. The purpose of research that compares differences in treatment or prescription rates between areas or organisations is usually to give the basis for further investigations into appropriateness of care. The purpose of comparing and combining studies of the same treatment in a meta-analysis is to establish the degree of certainty about effectiveness, or costs and benefits, which can be established from current knowledge or to compare economic calculations.

## Examples of comparative research within this category

Evaluations that compare treatments are described in detail in other texts (e.g. Pocock, 1983; Drummond et al., 1987; Fink, 1993; Øvretveit, 1998a). One example of a study into an illness-prevention treatment is a Swedish two-counties study of breast screening. This study found a 40% reduction in death from breast cancer in women who were offered mammography screening, compared to a control group who were not offered screening.

One of the earlier studies of international differences in surgical rates was that of McPherson et al. (1982). The study compared rates for common surgical procedures in New England, England and Norway, using data from hospital statistics which were reported to regional government or regional data centres, and standardised for age and sex. There have since been many similar studies and discussions of the validity of comparisons (e.g. Chassin et al., 1986; McPherson, 1989; Leape et al., 1990; Stano, 1993; Madsen, 1996).

# Service/health organisation comparisons

## Category definition

This category of research includes studies that compare health service teams, departments, hospitals and primary health care units. It also includes studies comparing purchasing or financing organisations, regulatory or inspection agencies, patient associations, professional associations and other health organisations.

A 'service' is here distinguished from a 'treatment', in that a service is one or more treatments carried out for a defined group of patients, or a health promotion service, project or programme. Most research in this category compares health care organisations, usually hospitals or specific hospital services (e.g. medical specialties). The category includes a growing number of information systems for routine performance comparisons, most of which are national or regional systems.

## Purposes of comparative research with this category

The purpose of many information systems within this category is to compare organisational performance or aspects of performance in order to contribute to managerial or policy actions and decisions. Some systems are designed to provide data to patients to help them choose a provider (Øvretveit, 1996a). Research studies, as distinct from routine information systems, involve more detailed data-gathering and analysis and often seek to explain differences in performance. Some research 'case study' comparisons aim to describe and explain differences in organisational characteristics, such as managerial structure and processes (e.g. Packwood et al., 1991).

## Concepts and issues

Studies within this category use different frameworks for comparison and different measures of performance. Performance comparisons are usually made in terms of:

- activity (e.g. number of patients treated, bed occupancy rate, bed turnover rates)

- costs/resource consumption (e.g. unit costs, bed day costs, DRG or equivalent costs)

- inputs/structure (e.g. number of staff, grade of staff, organisational roles and management structures)

- process (e.g. waiting times, quality indicators, satisfaction with 'hotel' facilities)

- outputs (e.g. the number of patients treated or personnel trained)

- outcome (e.g. mortality, morbidity and symptom reduction, satisfaction, resources used).

Within countries more time and resources are being devoted to develop comparative data about health service performance. In the UK there have been many revisions to the performance indicator dataset which has been running since the early 1980s (Appleby, 1993, 1996). In 1997 there were proposals in England to add clinical indicators such as death rates to the 70 indicators that are currently used to compile annual 'hospital league tables' (Walshe, 1997), and the 1998 NHS reforms have put a great emphasis on comparative performance measures.

There are lessons from this research and the discussions of the validity of comparative data for researchers in other fields. There are a number of issues to be considered in making performance comparisons, including:

- clearly defining the 'entity of measurement' and 'unit of performance' (e.g. exactly which service are we comparing? and when does, for example, a 'unit' of a patient-episode begin and finish?)

- which aspect of performance will we consider? (1) Economy: fewest resources or lowest cost (inputs), (2) Productivity: amount produced (output), (3) Efficiency: amount produced for the input (input/output), (4) Effectiveness: how well the service achieves the desired results (the change effected in the target; objectives met or needs/outcomes) or, (5) Quality: the degree to which the service satisfies patients, meets professionally assessed requirements, and uses the fewest resources within regulations (requirements met)

- the criteria the measures used to compare performance should meet:

  - The measures should help the people who gather the data to do their work better: which decisions should they be making which could be better informed by measures of their performance?

- Control: is the measure something which people can influence? (Do not measure what you can not do anything about)

- Process: is the measure related to a process (which people can describe and improve)?

- Three 'highs': high volume, cost and/or risk. Concentrate attention on measuring these

- Quick and easy to gather and use (ideally already collected)

- Credible: sufficiently reliable, valid and sensitive for the purpose and user

- Timely: least delay between event and presentation of measure (the 'Polaroid principle')

- Lowest cost/change: implementable using existing recording methods or computer systems, or with little change

- Politically acceptable: the collection and use of the measure will not change power balance between people in an unacceptable way.

## Service and organisation comparisons – examples

An example is a UK study that made a detailed comparison of hospital mortality in 22 London hospitals (Mckee & Hunter, 1995). The researchers used routinely reported in-hospital mortality rates and carried out adjustments by disease severity and on the basis of both admissions and episodes. The study then discussed issues and problems in producing and interpreting hospital mortality data, which also apply to other hospital outcome comparative data.

Another example of a study comparing hospital management structure was a comparison of the role of hospital medical directors in a sample of English hospitals (i.e. 'head of department'). The study involved interview and documentary data-gathering and produced descriptions of different roles and structures (IHSM, 1990). The concepts and discussion from this study have been used as a basis for comparing structures and the role of middle managers in Nordic hospitals.

# Comparisons of interventions to health organisations

## Category definition

This category of research includes studies that compare planned interventions to health organisations (typically hospitals), such as training or quality programmes, changes to structure, financing and new health personnel policies, such as reward and appraisal systems. Such studies consider interventions which have been made in one or a few organisations and compare these interventions either to 'no intervention' elsewhere, or to another intervention with a similar aim.

This category is different from the categories of 'health care reform' and 'health care policy' discussed below, even though many reforms and policies are also interventions to health organisations. The distinction is that 'interventions' to health organisations are of a specific type, usually only to a few organisations. Health care reforms or policies, on the other hand, usually involve a significant government-legislated change to all or many health organisations in a region and nation. Also, not all reforms and policies make changes to health organisations.

## Purposes of comparative research with this category

The purposes of comparing the same intervention in different organisations are to discover whether the intervention was introduced differently and whether it had different effects or costs. The purposes of comparing one or more organisations that underwent an intervention with those that did not is to assess the effects of the intervention and, sometimes, the costs. For these purposes it is common to select organisations that are similar in their context and in other features (e.g. the same country, same size, etc.), especially if the research takes an experimentalist perspective. This makes it possible to control or at least stabilise for influences other than the intervention, and thus to be more certain that any effects were due to the intervention. Many studies within this category use quasi-experimental or case study design and may be retrospective or prospective (*see* Chapter 5).

## Comparison of interventions to health organisations – examples

One example is a comparative case study of the quality programmes of six Norwegian hospitals (Øvretveit and Aslaksen, 1997, 1998). The study documented the quality programmes while they were being implemented, and described the experiences of each hospital on a number of dimensions. The researchers gathered data from middle managers about their experience and perceptions, using a standard semi-structured interview, and collated any evidence that was collected by the hospitals about the effects of the programmes. The study used a conceptual framework developed from previous research and from considering the aims of the quality programmes to compare the hospitals' experiences.

Other examples are comparisons of interventions to implement clinical practice guidelines in hospitals and primary care (Grimshaw *et al.*, 1995), and to implement integrated care pathways (Campbell *et al.*, 1998).

# Health system comparisons

## Category definition

This category of research includes studies which compare national and regional health service systems. 'Health system' is here defined as a collection of different health units which are organised and financed to provide a range of health services (often comprehensive) to a defined population or nation. Examples are national public health systems (e.g. UK, Icelandic and Italian), regional public systems (e.g. Scandinavian health systems) and private systems (e.g. Health Maintenance Organisations and Preferred Provider Organisations in the USA).

## Purposes of comparative research with this category

One purpose of making a comparison of national health systems is to discover differences and similarities in organisation, costs and effectiveness. A second purpose is to use this empirical knowledge to make improvements to the functioning of a health system or to contribute to scientific knowledge about the operation of complex systems within a larger context.

Some studies use a framework which defines different elements and aspects of performance of the system. This framework is used as a basis for cross-country or within-country data gathering and comparison (e.g. comparing elements such as the numbers of doctors, financing methods, extent of private ownership of facilities, inequalities, etc.). These frameworks are based on theories about the comparability of elements and about which features are significant for highlighting similarities and differences. Sometimes these frameworks involve theories about possible associations between variables, and often imply assumptions about relationships between the elements.

Some studies, usually those comparing a few countries, only have a general framework and define dimensions of similarity and difference during or after the data-gathering. These studies are more exploratory.

An example of one framework that is used for system comparison is the Nordic School of Public Health management programme, which compares national health systems in terms of: (a) 'input' or 'resource' indicators: cost per resident, doctors and nurses per 100 000, number of hospitals between 100 and 500, and 500 and 1000 beds, and other indicators; (b) 'structure and process': financing method, provider payment method, ownership, type of competition, regulatory methods, local autonomy and central powers, cost controls, incentives; and (c) 'patient performance': coverage, comprehensiveness, equity, choice, responsiveness, professional quality, health care and outcome indicators. (A useful collection of comparative essays on Nordic health systems is to be found in Alban & Christiansen, 1995.)

We can distinguish within this category two types of study. First, there are those which concentrate on one or a few aspects of health systems and aim to test hypotheses by comparing these aspects or variables across systems in different countries or within a country. A second type is the more comprehensive study which aims to describe the whole system as it functions and to make whole-system comparisons. Note, however, that it is often not possible to describe or compare a 'national health system' because of the great variety and differences within nations; in what sense can we speak of 'the' US health system? Consequently, in recent years there have been more cross-national comparisons of regional systems, or of one element across nations, although some comparisons of the latter type are of limited use without placing the element in context.

## Comparison of health systems – an example

A study which sought to overcome the problems of earlier system comparisons is that of Ellencweig (1992):

*If the various health systems were to converge, then they would be similar enough to permit their analysis by a simple unidimensional model. However, since convergence is not expected in the foreseeable future, we are left with a largely unsolved problem. How can we accurately compare systems, or assess different parts of a multisystem in a divergent, multidimensional environment?*

The answer given by this study is to divide a system and the elements to be compared into different 'modules', which include: population needs, resources, socio-economic development, organisation of health care and the process of health care delivery, health system outcomes and health outcomes. A 'macro-model' of a health system then proposes causal relationships between the modules.

The idea of this approach is that systems can be compared only in terms of one or more modules, where data are missing from some countries, or where some elements of the system are not comparable across countries. In the study, Ellencweig describes this framework and compares health systems, first by taking countries which were very different in relation to one of the modules but which were similar in others (Chapter 10) and second by taking three countries (Israel, Canada and Kenya) and attempting a whole-system comparison. The modular approach was used by Chinitz to compare reforms that increase competition within national health systems (Ellencweig, 1992).

## Health care reform comparisons

### Category definition

'Health care reform' is here defined as a significant change introduced by national or regional government legislation to the financing, organisation or functioning of health care services or to patients' rights. This category includes studies which compare the content, formulation and implementation of reforms to health care in different countries or regions in one country.

A 'reform' is different to a 'policy' in that, although policies often introduce changes, policies are usually more limited in scope and for specific purposes. However, some reforms (e.g. the Swedish 'personal doctor' reform of 1995) could equally be termed a new health policy. Note also that we are here making a distinction between reforms to health care service and health reforms (or health policies) which may not involve health care services (e.g. an environmental health reform or policy).

Some health care reforms involve multiple changes (e.g. the UK NHS reforms of 1991) and some make only one major change (e.g. the transfer from counties to municipalities in Sweden of responsibility for care of the elderly in 1992 – the 'Adel reforms'). There was a tendency in the early 1990s to view reforms as only market or internal competition reforms. Even though this type has been the most common type of reform in recent years, the category is broader than this. There is much that can be learnt from comparing market and non-market reforms; there are indications that some Swedish counties that have introduced restructuring and management development have increased efficiency more than those with purchaser-provider separation and market reforms.

## Purposes of comparative research with this category

The purpose of making comparisons of reforms to health care include:

- discovering the effects of similar reforms in different countries in order to make improvements or to predict the likely effects if it is introduced in one country

- examining how similar reforms have been introduced and differences in impact and 'absorption' in different situations

- helping policy-makers to formulate a reform and an implementation plan from the experience of others aiming to achieve a similar objective by their reform

- contributing to scientific knowledge about policy formulation and implementation.

The 1980s and 1990s were a period where many governments made or proposed health reforms and were influenced by reforms in other countries. Comparative research made a contribution to these reforms, and studies in the field drew on previous health systems comparisons. However, empirical data about the effects of reforms were not as plentiful or influential as theories and ideologies in both the academic and the policy debates. In part this was due to problems in comparison (Kroneman and van der Zee, 1997) and in researcher expertise. Overview comparisons include Ham *et al.* (1990), Ham (1997) and Saltman and Figuras (1997, 1998), and of Swedish counties reforms, Rehnberg (1997).

Since the early 1990s there has been an improvement in data and methodology, for example the OECD (1992) seven-country, and the OECD (1994) 17-country reforms comparisons. Other examples are the WHO European health reforms project and the International Clearinghouse of Health System Reforms Initiatives, the latter promoting comparative reform research and learning in developing countries (Block, 1997). There has also been an increasing number of single-study empirical comparisons, rather than separate research teams contributing reports to a standard format. An example of the former is the 'Eurobarometer' study which surveyed citizens of 15 European countries to gather data about their satisfaction with health care and their views about reforms and spending on health care (Mossialos, 1997).

## Comparison of health care reforms – an example

The WHO (1996b) comparison of health care reforms in Europe defined reform as 'a purposive, dynamic and sustained process that results in systematic structural change'. This study used a standard framework for researchers in each country to describe and assess changes to health care. It compared the pressures for reforms, different approaches to dealing with resource scarcity, equity in financing, resource allocation, efficiency in service delivery and different approaches to implementing reform. Part of the comparison also involved considering the context for implementation, the effects on and part played by primary care and patients' rights.

The WHO (1996b) report is part of a longer term programme which involves building a database and assessing the impact of reforms on health and in relation to the 'Health for all 2000' policy (WHO, 1981, 1992, 1994). This programme includes networks to collect and exchange information about reforms (e.g. 'MIDNET' for central Europe and 'CARNET' for central Asian republics) and 'Health Care System in Transition Profiles' (HiT) which gives detailed information about each country. Block (1997) discusses methods for comparative analysis of reforms in developing countries.

# Health policy and health care policy comparisons

## Category definition

This category of research includes studies which compare policies and laws to protect and improve health, as well as studies comparing policies applying to health care organisations.

## Purposes of comparative research with this category

The purposes of most comparative health policy research are to:

- describe policies in different countries and regions which have similar aims or content

- describe different policies which have achieved the same aims, or are intended to

- compare policy formulation or implementation processes or strategies.

The aims are to contribute to policy-making and implementation and to scientific knowledge about policy processes in government and society. Subfields within this category include international comparisons of policies and systems for prioritisation (e.g. Honingsbaum *et al.*, 1996) and on policies about patients' rights (e.g. Fallberg, 1996).

## Example of a comparative research study within this category

One subfield of comparative policy research is studies of policies to reduce inequalities in health status and in access to health care between regions or groups. One study described the health equality principles in Norway and Finland and their application in resource allocation methods (Samela, 1993). The study used national databases to compare patterns of distribution in the use of general hospital inpatient services in both countries, and regional differences in mortality and morbidity. The study discussed whether regional differences in the supply and use of health services are based on differences in need, and also considered possible future policy changes to reduce inequities.

## Conclusions

- Although having some methods and principles in common, comparative health research studies investigate many different subjects for a variety of purposes, and using many types of research approaches and methods.

- We can categorise types of comparative health research in terms of the subject and purpose of the research. Eight categories of studies are those comparing population health needs, health states and behaviour, treatments, health services and organisations, interventions to health organisations, health systems, health reforms, and both health policies and health care policies.

- By considering the range of studies we can learn about different methods that can help us to improve our own research. We can sometimes see the strengths, weaknesses, problems and potential of comparative studies in other people's research and then apply these insights to our own field of research.

- Appendix 4 gives a list of other example studies. More details of designs for different types of comparative research are given in Chapter 5 and of methods for data collection and analysis in Chapter 6.

# 3  Purposes, perspectives and philosophies

*Comparative health research is a broad field encompassing different research approaches with different purposes. There are also different philosophical assumptions underlying these approaches. Both researchers and users of research need to understand these differences in order to assess the value and use of a particular study.*

## Introduction

Chapter 2 showed the many types of comparisons that health researchers have made and showed some of the different methods used. We saw, for example, that we use different methods for an epidemiological comparison of disease to those we use to compare the implementation of policies to regulate nursing homes in different countries – a disease in a population is a different object of investigation to a policy implementation process.

One of the themes of this book is that there are concepts and principles which are common to all types of comparative research. Researchers from one field or discipline can learn from the solutions to problems of comparison developed by those working in another field. However, to learn from other fields and to carry out interdisciplinary research, we need to recognise different perspectives in research. In recent years, health research has come to include many different approaches. We need to understand the assumptions underlying other research approaches about the nature of reality and how to create valid knowledge about reality. In addition, users of comparative health research need to be aware of criteria for assessing the validity of a research study which are specific to a particular perspective, as well as the general criteria, which we consider in Chapter 4.

In this chapter we consider some of the different purposes and assumptions of comparative health research. We start by describing six different types: the descriptive, explanatory, experimental, phenomenological, genotypical and phenotypical. We then consider some of the philosophical assumptions underlying these different approaches and how studies conceptualise their object of investigation. The last part of the chapter shows a way to represent in a diagram the design used in a study. It shows how to represent the whole objects that are compared, the characteristic of those objects and the context 'surrounding' the whole object. It discusses the philosophical issues raised by this method of summarising a study.

Comparison is a powerful method for undertaking the two tasks of research – to describe and explain. Comparative research usually aims to:

- observe and describe (e.g. does the item exist in different places? What are the similarities and differences?)

- describe an association (e.g. is the presence or absence of an event or factor associated with the presence or absence of another event or factor in one place, and in different places?)

- establish causal mechanisms or influences (e.g. by making comparisons we can isolate possible influences and establish the evidence for and against one thing causing or influencing another)

- explain human action and perceptions in terms of both the meaning to the actors and the context (e.g. to explain, using comparisons, why people act differently in similar circumstances, or vice versa, or why a policy 'fails' in one place and 'succeeds' in another).

## Research approaches

We can describe a comparative health research study in terms of its purpose and research approach, characterised below as: descriptive, explanatory, experimental, phenomenological, genotypical and phenotypical. These are not mutually exclusive – a phenomenological approach may aim to both describe and explain.

## Descriptive

The aim of 'descriptive' comparative health research is either to discover whether or not an item or phenomenon is present in different places, or to describe the similarities and differences in comparable items. Examples of descriptive comparisons are:

- a description of GP remuneration systems in Australia, Canada, Denmark, Norway and the UK, which found large differences but also similarities between countries in the unclarity about the objectives of general practice (Kristiansen & Mooney, 1993)
- listing of health statistics in different countries (e.g. WHO, 1992; OECD, 1993b; NOMESCO, 1996, and other data comparisons)
- case study comparisons of health services or systems (which may or may not describe context).

Descriptive studies do not seek to explain the item or phenomenon which they discover or describe, but they may generate hypotheses or theories. Descriptive comparisons are made where there is little or no previous research and where the aim is to explore and document. In some studies, researchers seek to find whether an item found in one place can be found in others. Alternatively, researchers may suspect or know that the item or phenomenon does exist in different places and aim to describe it in more detail, and possibly also to explore how the item interacts with its context. This category of descriptive study does not, however, include descriptive 'observational' research, such as case–control comparisons or cohort studies: these are classified below as 'explanatory' (but not 'experimental') studies.

There are different types of descriptive comparative health research studies. 'Context-independent' studies seek to discover whether or not an item is present in different places, or how the item varies or differs between different places, but do not describe or consider the context (*see* Figure 3.2). 'Context-descriptive' comparisons describe both the item and its context in different places (*see* Figure 3.3). They may attempt to understand the items in terms of their different contexts, or may seek to find possible associations between variables or to generate explanatory hypotheses. Note that such 'comparative case studies' use different methods to those used in experimentalist studies (Yin, 1989).

'Level-oriented' descriptions compare the different level or magnitude of one variable in different places (e.g. differences in disease rates or differences in number of nurses). 'Structure-oriented' descriptive studies compare differences in the structure of an item between areas or in relationships among variables (e.g. do people have different sets of values or attitudes or are primary health care centres organised differently?).

# Explanatory

The aim of these studies is to explain the occurrence of a phenomenon or event by proving causation or by showing the probability of factors influencing the event. Explanation in some studies can also be in terms of providing an understanding or interpretation of an event or phenomenon in relation to its context. Examples are studies which:

- compare differences in death or disease rates and seek to explain the differences (e.g. cardiovascular mortality)

- consider why similarities in disease rates occur when theory suggests that the different conditions should result in different rates

- seek to explain differences in the way care is organised in different countries

- explain the success of a health policy in one place and its failure in another.

Some studies aim to explain the differences that can be found between comparable items which exist in different places, for example the different organisation of work in different health centres of similar size and services. Some studies aim to explain why items occur in one place but not another. Explanatory studies may use experimentalist or case-study methods, depending on the subject of comparison – case studies are more usual for health system and policy comparisons. Observational studies (e.g. 'case–control' studies) give less certain explanations than experimental studies, but are also used in comparative health research. Examples are studies that examine the history of people in one area who show a characteristic (cases) and compare their history with those of people in another area who do not show the characteristic (termed 'retrospective comparative case control' in Chapter 5).

Explanatory studies always consider context. They use comparison to discover whether context does or does not explain differences or similarities, or to discover which aspects of context are important. Many such studies seek to explain the presence, absence, amount or meaning of the item in different places by reference to differences in context and in how the item and context interact.

# Experimental

Experimental comparative health research introduces an intervention in one or more places to test a hypothesis. Such studies may introduce the same intervention in different places and examine the effects in these places, or they may introduce the intervention in one place and not in another and observe the effects. Alternatively, a study may treat an intervention such as a new policy as a 'natural experiment' and test hypotheses about effects and factors assisting the implementation. Experimental studies are always prospective: they are planned before the intervention is made. Some 'explanatory' studies are experimental or use experimentalist principles, as does a retrospective epidemiological case comparison study (sometimes termed an 'observational' study, as discussed in Chapter 5).

# Phenomenological

Phenomenological comparative research is a general category which describes research undertaken to understand and explain the meanings that people give to events. Much medical anthropological research falls into this category, and considers the different meanings that people in different cultures give to different health states. Phenomenological research is always descriptive, often explanatory and usually considers context. Some phenomenological research is termed 'qualitative research' or 'subjectivist' and builds up categories of meaning inductively out of the documented interviews or observations of the researcher (discussed at the end of Chapter 6).

# Phenotypical and genotypical comparisons

These terms refer not so much to a research perspective but to two different possible aims of a comparative study. Chapter 1 began by asking whether we could use scientific methods to improve our natural comparative abilities. In everyday life we often make superficial comparisons and assume that two things are different when closer examination shows them to have underlying similarities. I am not a gardening expert, but I am told that two plants that look different to me are in fact from the same plant family and are not really different at all. 'Genotypical' comparative health research is interested in discovering deep-level similarities in the phenomena in different areas, despite their superficial differences. The differences are due to the different environments in which organisms with the same genetic constitution have evolved. This term comes from biology, which defines 'phenotypical' differences as differences in outward appearances which are determined more by habitat than genes.

Another everyday error we make is to assume that two things are the same when further examination shows them to be different. Some comparative health research is interested in discovering deep-level differences in phenomena, despite their superficial similarities. For example, there may be a popular view that 'X' is the same, but further investigation shows that it is not (e.g. 'the' Nordic welfare model). By analogy with language, the same word can be used in different languages, but can mean different things. Research aiming to discover whether apparently similar items are different can be termed 'phenotypical comparative research'.

Note that whether something is the same or different in two places depends on which categories we use for comparison, not necessarily whether the thing is really the same or different. The notion used here is visual similarity – two things may 'look' the same, but if we use another way to compare them, they may be different. Note also that comparisons at a high level of abstraction tend to show similarities, and that the more

---

**Box 3.1: Summary of research approaches**

*Descriptive CHR*: research to discover the presence or absence of an item in different places or to describe similarities and differences (e.g. statistical comparisons, some survey comparisons, some case studies)

*Explanatory CHR*: research that aims to understand, interpret or explain why similarities or differences occur (e.g. many epidemiological studies, some case studies)

*Experimental CHR*: aims to test a hypothesis by intervening in one or more places and by using statistical methods to establish the probability of the hypotheses being true or false (e.g. a controlled trial)

*Phenomenological CHR*: seeks to understand and interpret the meanings that people give to events and experiences in different cultures or places (e.g. the reactions and coping strategies of people diagnosed with cancer in different ethnic groups)

*Genotypical CHR*: research interested in discovering deep-level similarities in the phenomena in different areas or countries, despite the apparent differences between the phenomena ('the items look different, but there are underlying similarities')

*Phenotypical CHR*: research that examines superficially similar items to discover deep-level differences ('the items looks the same, but there are underlying differences')

detailed the comparison, the more likely we are to find differences. The health systems of Norway and Sweden appear the same at a high level of abstraction – they are both financed out of taxation and locally governed, but if we look in more detail the differences become more apparent. For example, there are different co-payment rates, proportions of public and private services, and differences in governance at commune, county, regional and national levels.

# Perspectives and assumptions underlying a comparative study

*The basis of all science is observation, but the beginning of observation is categories which allow perception. Without categories which draw boundaries between one thing and another, we cannot perceive the world. Comparison allows us to see differences and to create categories. Comparative research has an important contribution to make to science because it gives us a method for constructing and critically examining our concepts of the world.*

How we assess the validity of a comparative study depends on our assumptions about what constitutes a fact and what we mean by a scientific explanation. These assumptions are also the basis for how a researcher plans and conducts a study. We consider these assumptions in more detail here, for two reasons. First, there are some criteria of validity that are specific to studies carried out within a particular perspective. Comparisons made using an 'experimentalist' perspective have to meet criteria for controlling variables and hypothesis testing which are not required in 'subjectivist' perspectives that study phenomena in their 'real-life' context. Chapter 4 describes six sets of general criteria for planning and assessing the validity of a comparative study, but we note below that there are also specific criteria for different perspectives and why this is so.

A second reason is that it is important that researchers and users of research are aware of the philosophical assumptions underlying the comparison made in a particular study and of their own assumptions. One of the many interesting aspects of comparative research is how it makes us aware of these assumptions. When we make a comparison, are we comparing two or more real things or just our concepts of these things? This is one of the questions that we consider in this short discussion of philosophical assumptions.

# Ontology and epistemology

Each comparative study makes assumptions about the nature of their object of study (ontology), and about how to gain valid knowledge about that object (epistemology). Each study has assumptions about the purpose of science and about which type of descriptive and explanatory statements are acceptable (i.e. what counts as facts, data or evidence).

Empiricist assumptions are that an item has an independent objective reality separate from the observer, and that this will reveal itself to the observer if they observe carefully and objectively. Careful observation will allow the researcher to construct categories which reflect the reality. These assumptions are often associated with experimental or epidemiological research and with studies that gather quantitative data, but not all research takes such a simple view. Also, note that some research using qualitative methods to gather data about people's views or their reflections on their experience is empiricist. It is empiricist because it assumes that people have views and ideas already formed and they simply transpose these on to a questionnaire or verbalise their pre-existing ideas in an interview. Yet it is common for people not to have given any thought to the subject they are being questioned about, and the method of data-gathering itself helps the person create their views. The data-gathering method is not neutral or a simple medium for pre-existing data, but creates and shapes the data.

Most research that can be described as 'positivist' and 'subjectivist' is empirical in the sense that it involves data-gathering. Yet much of this research is not based on empiricist assumptions because it recognises that concepts and theories are necessary for the researcher to gather data in the first place. (Note also that 'non-empirical comparative research' is research that does not involve data-gathering and which is concerned only with methodological or conceptual construction and theoretical analysis.) Table 3.1 summarises these three philosophical perspectives of empiricist, positivist and subjectivist, and the views about facts and explanation which characterise each.

If positivist studies involve the empirical collection of data, but they are not empiricist in their assumptions, then what are the assumptions held by such studies about reality and facts? Positivism also holds that the world has an objective reality independent of the observer. But unlike simple empiricism it recognises that we cannot study this reality without first having some concepts to guide our observations. Positivism takes the view that reality can be apprehended through pre-observational categories, and that we continually improve our representations of reality through refining our categories and by testing hypotheses derived from theories.

**Table 3.1**: Different views about evidence and explanation in comparative health research

| Philosophical perspective | What are facts? | How to collect data | What is an explanation? | What is the aim of science? |
|---|---|---|---|---|
| *Empiricist* | Facts are what we observe | Objective observation and measurement | Facts speak for themselves | Collect facts which describe the world |
| *Positivist* | With pre-observational categories, we can gather data empirically to refute hypotheses | Objective observation and measurement. Objectivity lies in the researcher's detachment from the subject of study, their value neutrality and in the accuracy of data collection | Showing association between variables. Showing the probability of one variable influencing another. Seeking causal explanations. Describing the laws governing phenomena | Test hypotheses derived from theories. By seeking to falsify hypotheses, increase the certainty of explanatory statements and gradually build up knowledge |
| *Subjectivist* | Facts are a person's or group's subjective understanding of an event, or the meaning and value which they give to their experience | Participant observation, interviewing. The validity of data lies in the ability of the researcher to fully enter into and empathise with the subjects' perception and experience, and their ability to represent this authentically | Understanding an act or phenomenon by reference to the meaning of the event for the actor and to the rules which give that act meaning | To explain actions and social events by reference to the values and meanings of those involved and by reference to social rules followed by subjects |

Objectivity lies in the researcher's detachment from the object of study, their value neutrality and in the accuracy of data collection. Data can be thought of as being more or less adequate representations of a reality which exists independently of the researcher's methods and concepts.

In natural sciences, this approach views physical objects as being subject to law-like processes which can be discovered, and uses causality to explain events. These assumptions are applied both to physical objects or processes such as disease in the human body, and to social objects such as organisations and policies. In the latter, we can find causes and law-like regularities in human action and social objects without referring to people's perceptions or values: the objects studied are governed by causes whether or not people are aware of them.

Underlying some comparative research studies of social entities and processes are a different set of assumptions, which we can term 'subjectivist' (sometimes termed 'phenomenological' or 'constructivist'). This approach holds that people, both individually and in groups, are not determined by causal factors, but attribute meaning to the physical and social world. People have choice and create their own worlds and actions. Their actions and the 'shape' of social organisations and policies cannot be understood without reference to the meanings and values of the people involved in their creation and recreation. Researchers who see people's meanings and values as important to understanding social phenomena use data-gathering methods and designs which give access to these meanings. The validity of data depends on the ability of the researcher to fully enter into and empathise with the subject's perception and experience, and their ability to represent this 'authentically'.

These approaches have different ways of conceptualising their object of study and its relation to its context. A positivist and experimentalist perspective views the item studied as having an objective reality independent of the observer and their measuring instrument. The perspective seeks to explain the relationship between the item and context in causal terms – to identify factors that have a causal influence independent of the perceptions of the human beings involved. A subjectivist perspective investigates people's perceptions of the relationship between the context and the item. Explanations are in terms of how factors are perceived to influence the item, and meanings.

The next part of the chapter shows a general method for representing the object of a comparative study and the context of the object. We will see that, while the same model can be used to represent all comparative studies, studies differ in how they conceptualise the object and its relation to its context. The diagrams illustrate and further discuss these philosophical assumptions underlying comparative studies.

# A diagrammatic model for representing a comparative research study

A diagram is a simple but effective way for quickly making sense of and summarising a research study. One indication of an overcomplex or poor design is that it is difficult to draw a diagram of the study. The diagram should show:

- the *whole objects* that are compared (e.g. populations, organisations, policies)

- the *characteristics* of the whole objects that are compared (e.g. death rates in different populations, the organisation of primary care centres, training programmes in different hospitals)

- the *context* surrounding the item compared (described in terms of the factors which may have an effect on the compared item (causality) or which may affect the meaning of the item (interpretation), such as economic, historical, political or cultural contexts).

Figure 3.1 shows the 'basic model' of a research study: it shows just one of the 'whole objects' to be compared, for example a hospital, and the context

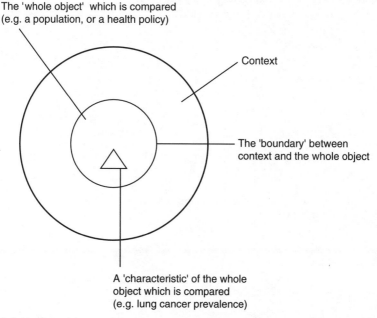

**Figure 3.1** Basic model.

could include the financial and competitive environment. The 'whole object' could also be a process, such as the implementation of a health policy reform, and the context could be political and other factors that may affect the process.

A comparative study does not compare whole objects as such, but compares characteristics of the objects, such as death rates or organisation. Similarly, the study will not compare contexts as such, but will conceptualise characteristics of the context which are compared, such as the amount of crime in a community or the degree of competition for labour or referrals.

## A simple comparison (context not considered; Figure 3.2)

Figure 3.2 shows a simple comparison that does not consider the context of the items which are compared. The whole object is the sample of a population and the disease is the characteristic which is compared. This diagram illustrates the point that it is not the whole objects that are compared, but one or more characteristics. The triangle shown inside the whole object represents this characteristic (the disease) of the whole object (the population). The diagram represents a study which aims to answer the question 'is there any difference in the prevalence of this disease between two areas?'

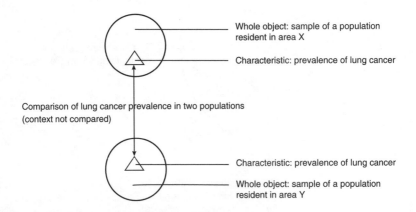

Figure 3.2 'Item comparison' (e.g. for descriptive comparisons)

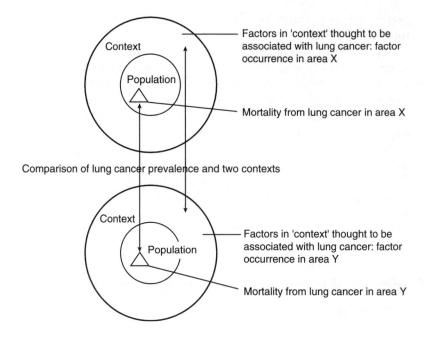

**Figure 3.3** 'Item and context comparison' (e.g. for explanatory comparisons)

## Context and item comparison (Figure 3.3)

Figure 3.3 can be used to represent a study that describes and compares both the item and the context in both areas. This diagram shows a comparison of the characteristic of the population, and also a comparison of the context. The study would define different aspects of the context of each population which are theorised as possibly relevant for explanation or understanding, for example housing conditions or cultural factors such as religious beliefs.

## How to use the models

Readers of a comparative study can use these models to draw a simple diagram of the study. This helps to understand the main features and show what is compared. Researchers will also find a diagram is a powerful way of presenting their study simply and of helping others to see the key features of the design.

The diagram can also be used to show how strongly the whole object is influenced by the context. A dotted line encircling the whole object shows that the boundary between the object and context is not clearly demarcated and shows an interaction between object and context. The diagrams are also useful for raising questions about whether the boundaries are real or conceptual boundaries.

A more detailed diagrammatic representation would show the study over a period of time, with a time line at the bottom of the diagram and an indication of the times at which data were collected. The research designs described in Chapter 5 can be represented in diagrammatic form (*see* Øvretveit, 1998a, Chapter 3).

## Conceptual boundaries and philosophical assumptions

The 'basic model' above (Figure 3.1) shows the 'whole object' separated from its 'context' by a 'boundary', and Figures 3.2 and 3.3 represent different types of comparative study designs. But is the boundary between the object and context real, or is it just a conceptual boundary? For example, when comparing hospital organisational structures we define a hospital as the 'whole object'. But where do the boundaries of the hospital end? Are the boundaries real or conceptual constructions, or both? What is the nature of the 'whole objects' compared, such as people, populations, institutions and policies, and how do we create valid descriptive and explanatory knowledge about such objects? We now consider the assumptions that different studies make about the nature of the item and its relationship with the context.

If we take account of the assumptions of different research perspectives discussed earlier, we need to add to these models the way in which a particular study relates the item studied to its context – through causality or other types of influences, such as system dynamics. Some studies do not start with a clear definition of the boundary between the item and context, but this might not necessarily be bad research: the study may, through comparison, develop a clear boundary definition of the item.

If we recognise the philosophical assumptions underlying a research study we can see that different studies have a different answer to the following questions: do the 'items' we compare really exist or are they the constructions of our concepts and research procedures? Is 'suicide' an objective fact or something created by our categories and data-gathering methods? It even leads us to question what a study means by 'death' – is it a real event or something created through a concept of death? It is both – the approach taken in this book views facts as created in an interaction between the researcher and reality, and in a social interaction between researchers that defines which methods will be used to agree what is a fact and what is an adequate explanation. One of the values of a comparative approach is to highlight some of these assumptions.

## The item boundary, interaction and stability

Given the different philosophical assumptions behind different types of comparative research, we can see why studies differ in terms of how they conceptualise their objects of study: the 'whole object', its character-istics and the context. We now describe these different assumptions. The main differences are in how the research defines the item, whether the item changes and how it interacts with its environment.

### ITEM BOUNDARY DEFINITION: CLEAR OR FUZZY BOUNDARY DEFINITION

Some comparative research clearly defines the item (i.e. either the whole object or one or more of its characteristics) to be compared; the boundary between the item and its context is clearly defined (*see* Figure 3.1). An example is research into a disease (a characteristic of a population, the population being the 'whole object'), where there is a generally accepted operational definition of the disease which allows its easy identification and discrimination from other diseases.

Some comparative research, on the other hand, does not make a clear boundary definition between the item and its context. Indeed the aim of the research may be to identify and define a phenomenon which is thought to have a distinct existence, such as a hospital quality programme, and to do so by making comparisons.

Note that we are not making any assumptions about the reality which the research seeks to describe; we are describing the way in which the research defines its objects of study. We are describing the research, not reality. Neither are we making any judgements about the quality of the research. It may be that other researchers have made a clearer definition of the object and have shown that the item can be clearly differentiated from its context and from other items. If so, then we may consider that the study makes a 'poor' definition of its object if it has not considered this previous research. Note also that the research might start with a 'fuzzy' boundary definition and conclude with a 'clear' boundary definition; the purpose may be to find through comparative research whether a clear boundary definition can be made (e.g. do the things which people describe as a 'hospital quality programme' have something in common?).

INTERACTION BETWEEN THE ITEM AND CONTEXT

This refers to how the research conceptualises the relationship between the item and its context: does it consider the item (e.g. a disease or a hospital quality programme) to be unaffected or strongly influenced by factors in the environment? Does the research assume, or conclude, that the item is unaffected or relatively unaffected by its context, or is in constant inter-action with its context? For example, many comparative studies of cancer mortality examine whether different mortality rates might be associated with different environmental factors. A study may test the null hypothesis that one factor has no effect, but it does so to test the theory that cancer mortality may be affected by this environmental factor. Again, note that we are not making any assumptions about reality: about whether the item is really strongly or little affected by context. We are just describing the assumptions or how the research presents its findings.

We can use different terms and metaphors to describe how the research conceptualises the interaction, or lack of it, and the type of boundary. 'Concrete boundary' suggests that the item is isolated from and unaffected by context. A 'permeable boundary' suggests that the context affects the item, but also that the item can affect the context: a two-way interaction. A 'symbiotic relationship' suggests a mutual interdependence between item and context. Finally, 'osmosis' suggests a specific type of relationship between context and the item, where the item is thought of as being like a concentrated solution separated from a less concentrated solution (the 'context') by a semi-permeable boundary. The influence is one-way from the context to the item, but is a particular type of influence: the flow is of a less concentrated solvent of the dissolved molecules (in the 'context') through the 'membrane' boundary into a more concentrated solution (the 'item') until both context and item are the same concentration.

ITEM STABILITY AND DYNAMICS

A third way of describing a research study is in terms of how it con-ceptualises the stability of the item it studies. If this is not explicit, what are the study's assumptions about the stability or changing nature of the item?

An item such as mortality can be described as stable in the sense that death is not usually conceptualised as something that changes: it is or it is not. Thus comparisons of mortality are comparisons of a stable item. An item such as a hospital may be viewed as stable for certain purposes of comparison, for example a comparison of management structures at one time. Examples of studies that compared items which changed over time are a study of the implementation of resource management in six hospitals (Packwood *et al.*, 1991) and a study of quality programmes in different hospitals over five years (Øvretveit & Aslaksen, 1998).

# Conclusions

- Health research that involves comparisons is a category of research which includes studies of many different subjects, such as diseases, organisations and policies. Different methods are used to study different subjects, but there are some concepts, methods and principles which apply to all comparative research.

- The aim of some comparative studies is description and exploration. Many such studies aim to find out if an item exists in other places, or the similarities and differences in comparable items in different places.

- Some comparative research aims to explain why similarities or differences occur. Such research often uses experimentalist methods and tests hypotheses.

- Subjectivist or phenomenological comparative research can also involve hypothesis testing, but aims to understand and interpret the meanings which people give to events and experiences in different places.

- Some comparative research is interested in discovering whether there are deep-level similarities between items in different places which appear different ('genotypical' comparative research), or whether items which appear the same are different in other respects ('phenotypical' comparative research).

- A valid comparison does not have to compare similar things: a valid comparison can be made between items which appear different if the aim is to find out if there are any deep-level similarities ('genotypical research').

- A diagram of a comparative study is a good way to summarise it. Such a diagram should show the items that are compared: the whole objects, the characteristics and whether the context is considered.

- Comparative studies differ in terms of how they conceptualise their subject and in the assumptions they hold about the stability of the item compared and its interaction with its context.

# 4    Making true comparisons

*How can a user of a research study decide if the comparisons and conclusions of the study are valid? How can a researcher ensure that their study makes valid comparisons? How can a research supervisor or financier assess a proposal for comparative research?*

## Concepts for assessing or planning a comparative research study

The methodological problems involved in comparative health research are greater than in many other types of research. Concepts and their operational definitions may be different in different areas, but we may not notice the difference and thus make comparisons which are not valid. Bias is the deviation of collected data from a 'true value' or the 'true perception' of a subject who is interviewed, and is introduced by data-gathering methods not being applied consistently. Data bias is a problem in most comparative research, for example when we use already-collected data, such as national health statistics. This chapter considers issues of validity and reliability in general terms for all kinds of comparative study and also gives a background for Chapters 5 and 6, which look at design and data gathering in more detail.

The chapter gives six sets of criteria for assessing whether a study makes valid comparisons and produces true and useful conclusions. Researchers planning a study will also find these criteria helpful for making decisions about research design, data-gathering methods and other matters. One theme is that we can only assess the methods used in a study in relation to the question or problem which the study addresses. This chapter proposes that the validity of a comparative research study depends on:

1 the quality of the research problem statement, question or hypothesis

2 the validity of the comparisons made in the study

3 the validity of the research design for the purpose of the research (the ability of the design to answer the question; more details are given in Chapter 5)

4 the validity of the data-gathering methods and the quality of the data which were gathered (discussed in detail in Chapter 6)

5 the validity of the data analysis

6 the justification for the conclusions and the logical connections through-out the report.

To some extent this list corresponds to the steps involved in carrying out a research study. We will see that the validity of the conclusions are only as good as the weakest of these steps and depends on the chain of reasoning which links each part. Appendixes 2 and 3 give a full checklist of questions for assessing a study.


# I Defining the research question or hypothesis

*In everyday life we make comparisons because we cannot help doing so. In science we make comparisons for a specific purpose: to test a hypothesis or to answer a question. Without this specific purpose, a comparison which is 'open ended' is likely to be inconclusive and wasteful of both the researcher's and other people's time.*

A study that aims to 'contribute to knowledge by comparing 'X' in different countries' is not likely to produce useful conclusions unless this aim is later restated as a more specific question or hypothesis to be tested. What exactly do the researchers mean by 'X' and how will data be gathered about 'X'? How will data about 'X' in different places contribute to knowledge – just by adding to the data mountain, or by helping to resolve controversies, filling important gaps in knowledge or by testing conflicting theories?

The research question is the engine and the compass for a research study. It gives the motivation and direction to all subsequent steps by defining the significance of the research and by delimiting and focusing the work. Poorly stated and vague research questions are entirely appropriate for a wandering and wasteful research project.

There needs to be a well-defined and specific question, problem statement or hypothesis (depending on the type of study), with a rationale for taking a comparative approach. This needs to follow from a review of knowledge which shows how the research will fill a gap or how it builds on previous research. There also needs to be significance and value: would an investigation of this question or hypothesis be of interest and make a difference to the world?

It takes time, skill and knowledge of the field to define a fruitful research question or testable hypothesis, and doing so is, in my view, the most important part of a research study because nearly everything else flows from this. It is also the part of the research which is most often neglected, especially by inexperienced researchers in their eagerness to start collecting data. Perhaps the most valuable contribution which a research supervisor or advisor can make is to help a researcher work on and focus their question or hypothesis.

We can talk of the 'validity' of the research question or the hypothesis, not in the sense of truth or untruth, but in the sense of the question or hypothesis 'having authority' and being significant. This depends first on whether it relates to previous research and could help move knowledge forward or fill a gap and, second, on who might use or be interested in the results of such research and what difference the knowledge could make to them and the world. 'Who cares?': if there is no immediate and obvious answer to this after reading the research question or hypothesis, then one must wonder whether the research is more for the benefit of the researchers than for practical or scientific purposes, and whether their time and effort might be put to better use.

Significance is one way to judge the quality of the research question in a study. The other and more conventional way is in terms of whether the question is well defined in the sense of being clear, specific and answerable, or whether the hypothesis is testable. Users of research with little time would be advised to start their reading of a paper by looking for the research question. If they cannot find one or if it is unclear or trivial, then they should think twice before reading further.

There are no simple guidelines for how to define a fruitful research question and surprisingly little written on such an important topic, but there are criteria which have been suggested. Kerlinger (1986), working within a positivist tradition, proposes criteria for a 'good' research problem statement or hypothesis: (i) Does the statement express a relationship between variables? (ii) Is it capable of being empirically tested? (iii) Is it stated in unambiguous terms in a question form?

In similar vein, Open University (OU, 1973) proposes five criteria for assessing a research problem statement: (i) Does it state relationships between variables? (ii) Is it 'testable' or 'resolvable' in terms of making a prediction or having a possibility of answering the question? (iii) Is it limited in scope and realistic? (The more global the statement, the less likely it will be to confirm or refute it. Only a limited study can produce significant findings, but some studies produce trivial findings.) (iv) Is the statement not inconsistent with most known facts? (v) Is it stated clearly with indications of how abstract variables will be operationalised?

The latter criterion brings us back to the point about the importance of a research question in giving a direction and focus to a study. This criterion proposes that the problem statement should include an indication of the measures which will be used or how the abstract concept (e.g. health, quality programme) is to be operationalised. This refers to both how the dependent and independent variables, or the aspects of context and the conceptual comparison, are to be operationalised. The point here is that the research question can be made more precise and the research more focused by the researcher considering how to gather data which will refute, confirm or allow exploration of the concepts. For example, take a researcher's or sponsor's general idea of comparing the effects of a policy in two different countries: the research statement can be made more precise by considering what would constitute evidence of effects of this policy and how could we gather data which would be accepted as evidence.

The above criteria can be used to assess the 'quality' of a research problem statement, but researchers working within a phenomenological tradition might find them too restrictive, and as implying one model of research. Note that hypothesis testing is also an important technique in, for example, historical comparisons or anthropological or ethnographic studies: stating hypotheses helps to focus a study and can help researchers to define their assumptions before data gathering. However, the emphasis above on defining the question is not intended to suggest that researchers never change their question or hypothesis as the research proceeds. In some types of research this is necessary and part of the research process. It is intended to suggest that the report should describe the starting question, the changes that were made and why.

# Practical guidelines for defining the purpose of the research and the problem statement

How then should a researcher define the right research question? Can a user of comparative research judge whether to read a study just by looking at the research question? There are no simple answers to these questions, but the following gives some guidance and criteria. I have found that answering the following questions is helpful in defining the purpose of my own and others' research:

- who is the research for? (who are the 'users' of the research?)
- what do they want or need to know?
- why do they want or need to know this? (how could they act differently if they knew this?)
- why is a comparative study necessary to discover this?

Two sets of criteria for formulating or assessing a research question were noted above. In my view they are useful for experimental research, but less useful for some policy and case-study comparisons. The criteria in Box 4.1 apply to all types of comparative health research.

---

**Box 4.1: Assessing the quality of the research question or hypothesis – summary checklist**

- Did the study sufficiently consider previous research and draw on this to define the question or the hypothesis?
- Does the study give a clear and specific question which is answerable, or a testable hypothesis?
- Is the question or hypothesis to be tested significant, of interest and likely to help people make better-informed decisions?
- Does the study give a justification for the cost and efforts of a comparative study rather than another type of study?

---

# 2 Validity of the comparison

*Some cross-national and cross-cultural comparisons are not valid because they impose a concept which only has meaning in one area or culture on others, or do not recognise differences in the meaning of concepts between areas or cultures.*

The validity of the comparison made by a study depends on three things, whether:

(i) the different populations, institutions, processes or other 'whole objects' which are compared are in fact comparable for the purposes of the research (the validity of the 'whole object comparison'; Figure 3.1 in the last chapter shows the 'whole object')

(ii) the conceptual comparison is valid: whether it is valid to compare the particular aspects or characteristics of the 'whole objects' which are compared (the validity of the 'conceptual comparison'; *see* Figure 3.2)

(iii) the concepts are operationalised in a valid way in the data-gathering method or measure, and whether the same operational concepts are used in all the areas where data are gathered.

We will consider (iii) later when we look at how to assess the data-gathering methods used in a study. The differences between these three types of validity are illustrated by the example of comparing suicide in the Nordic countries. The 'whole object comparison' of different populations is valid in general terms, but the validity would also depend on the question or hypothesis to be tested and the sample used. Comparing suicide rates is also a valid 'conceptual comparison' because the concept of suicide is comparable between the Nordic countries. However, because different countries have different ways of registering death as suicide or accident for national data gathering (NOMESCO, 1996, p. 124), a comparison of suicide rates from these statistics would be an invalid comparison if there was no adjustment for these differences.

'Whole object' comparability refers to two things. First, how particular populations, institutions or other items in different places are chosen and the validity of the selection (sampling). Second, in some studies it refers to the concept of the whole object – for example how the subject defines 'policy implementation process' or 'hospital' and whether this concept is comparable across areas; some countries classify hospitals as a single building on one site with over 10 beds, whereas other countries define a hospital differently.

'Conceptual comparability' refers to whether the characteristic or variable of the item studied in area X is the same or comparable to that studied in area Y and other areas. 'Conceptual comparability' does *not* refer to how the concept is operationalised for data gathering, and whether this is done in the same way in data gathering in different places (i.e. the third criterion above).

In many types of comparative research a comparison is made between whole objects in terms of one or more characteristics or variables which are defined before data gathering. The research needs to show that it is meaningful and valid to compare the 'whole objects' in terms of this one or more characteristics or variables. In research that asks questions of the general public we need to consider the comparability of the concept, for example in terms of the typical person's understanding of it. This is referred to as 'concept equivalence'. For example, 'headache' means something different to the typical Norwegian than it does to the typical Australian Aborigine. When we are asking questions of the general public 'conceptual equivalence' is an important issue, and a different and prior question to how well the concept is operationalised or translated in a questionnaire.

Conceptual comparability is essential for research which defines concepts before data gathering, but not for all types of comparative research. Some exploratory research aims to discover how people understand the meaning of a concept in two or more populations or cultures. Some examine whether there are deeper-level differences in apparently similar phenomena. In these types of research the aim is to build up concepts from the subjects' views and to discover similarities and differences, rather than to start with precisely pre-defined concepts. Thus, some comparative research studies can be valid even if they do not involve comparable concepts: the research may aim to find out if a concept in one area has meaning in another area, or whether comparable concepts can be found in subject populations, or the differences in meaning of the concept in different areas or cultures.

'Comparability' does not mean that the item or the concept has to be exactly the same in all the areas studied. The research may investigate an item that appears similar, to find out if there are any deeper-level differences (phenotypical research), or one that appears different, to find out if there are any deeper-level similarities (genotypical research). Thus some comparative research does not assume concept comparability; rather it seeks to discover whether two events, items or phenomena are really similar, regardless of whether or not they appear to be. In this instance the research is not made less true or invalid if the research discovers that apparently similar items are in fact different.

---

**Box 4.2: Concept comparability – summary checklist**

- Does the research define the whole object and the characteristic(s) of it which are to be compared in different areas?

- Does the research consider the possible reasons for items in different areas not being comparable?

- If the research involves data gathering from subjects, does the study adequately justify using the same concept in different populations if the concept does not have the same meaning to subjects in these different populations?

# 3 Validity of the design for the purpose

To assess the validity of the design we need to ask whether the design chosen was one that could answer the research question or test the hypothesis. Design validity depends on:

- valid sampling (the size, type and location of the sample)

- what is compared (the concept)

- how often, when and over which time period the data are gathered in different places

- whether the data-gathering and analysis methods are suited to both the nature of the subject studied and to the research question

- how all the above are linked to the research question.

Strictly speaking an assessment of the design should be done after assessing the concept comparability and the data-gathering methods. However, when assessing or planning a study it is useful to consider the suitability of the design in general terms, before then looking at the details of data gathering and analysis and at other details of design.

Both the conceptualisation of the item compared (discussed above) and the data-gathering methods are part of the design, but in this account we have considered these separately. Chapter 5 describes different designs and considers which is best for different purposes. Methods to enhance validity that are used before the data collection are called 'a priori' procedures and those used after data collection 'a posteriori' procedures.

---

**Box 4.3: Design quality – summary checklist**

- Is there a clear description of the items to be compared, the timescale and other aspects of design?

- Are there too few or too many items compared in order to answer the research question or test the hypothesis?

- In practice, is the design practical and capable of being carried out by reasonably well-trained researchers with the amount of resources that could be expected for this type of study?

- In theory, is the sample and the design able to answer the research question or test the hypothesis, if the study is carried out perfectly?

# 4 Validity of the data-gathering method and of the data

This refers mainly to the validity and reliability of the data-gathering methods, both for a single population or site study and for a multiple population or site comparative study. Questions to ask to assess the data-gathering method are:

- will the method gather data that will help answer the research question?
- is the method a valid and reliable one for gathering data about the subject?
- how was the method used in different places or for different populations?

First we consider validity and then reliability.

## Validity of the data-gathering method

In most types of research the validity of the data-gathering method refers to whether the method could produce data which 'truly reflects' the characteristics of the 'whole object' or the concept studied. For example, does a measure of the 'performance' of a hospital really measure performance, or something else? Does the Hamilton Depression Scale really gather data about 'depression' or about something else?

This type of validity is often termed 'construct validity' and refers to whether the operationalisation of the concept measures what it is intended to measure. In comparative research it is possible that a data-gathering method is valid in one culture or country but not in another. Thus we have to be concerned about construct validity in all the places or populations where the measure is used. This is easier if we use a standard measure or method of data gathering, and where research has already been carried out to assess the validity of the method in the type of places or populations studied.

The most common ways of assessing the validity of a data-gathering method in one place or population are:

- *Face validity*: the data-gathering method appears to measure what it claims to measure (a simple test of face validity is to ask someone knowledgeable about the phenomenon if they think the measure represents the phenomenon).

- *Criterion validity*: the data-gathering method or measure produces data that correlate with data from another method which is accepted as a valid measure of the thing studied (i.e. its consistency with alternative measures or data-gathering methods).

- *Predictive validity*: the ability of the method to predict an event.

- *Content validity*: the measure comprehensively covers the things it is intended to measure (e.g. a quality-of-life measure covers all aspects of quality of life or an exam covers all of a course – often linked to a conceptual model of the thing being measured). In comparative research we sometimes find that a survey designed in one culture does not comprehensively cover the items it needs to cover in another culture to capture data about the same phenomenon.

If a method is found valid in one place according to these tests, the same tests need to be applied to the use of the method in the other places or populations where the comparison is made.

## Reliability of the data-gathering method and of the data

This refers to whether the method is able to produce consistent data and to whether the methods were applied consistently in different places or populations. It is mainly concerned with how the method is administered. There are three commonly used concepts of reliability:

- *Inter-rater reliability*: the extent to which two or more observers give the same value to the thing they measure.

- *Intra-rater reliability*: the same observer gives the same value at different times, if the thing he or she observes is the same.

- *Stability*: of a measure refers to its ability to give the same scores at different times if nothing has changed (this is sometimes called 'test-retest reliability').

The reliability of the data refers to the amount of random or systematic error (bias) or variance in the data, either between times (e.g. one interviewer at different times) or between units (e.g. between interviewers or target populations). A measure may be unreliable because it is difficult for the subject to understand (e.g. ambiguous questions) or because the setting or method of administration affects the measure (e.g. a hospital patient is given a satisfaction questionnaire by a nurse and asked to return it to the nurse).

As we see in Chapter 5, data from interviews can sometimes be unreliable. Unless certain precautions are taken, such as careful training, different interviewers may elicit and collect different data. This is not to suggest that qualitative data are always less reliable than quantitative data.

To finish this discussion of how to assess the data-gathering methods and data in a comparative study, we need to note two other criteria.

## Sensitivity and specificity

'Sensitivity' describes the ability of a method to correctly identify a thing or an event, such as a disease or a person with a particular characteristic, it is how well the measure detects the health problem or thing it is intended to measure (sometimes termed 'responsiveness'). A measure such as a test for anxiety could be valid for two ethnic groups but may only detect high levels of anxiety in one of the groups.

'Specificity' describes how well a measure identifies people without a particular health problem or who do not exhibit the characteristic

---

**Box 4.4: Data-gathering methods and data quality – summary checklist**

- Are the data-gathering methods appropriate for answering the question or the hypothesis to be tested? For a study of this type in *one* place, are the methods suitable for gathering data about a subject of this type?

- Does the research use valid operational definitions of the concept(s)?

- Are the operational definitions the same for *all* the data gathering, in different areas or populations?

- Are all possible differences considered in how the data were collected in different places or for different populations?

- Were the precautions adequate for ensuring that the data were collected in the same way in different places or populations? (The reliability of the method for the comparison)

- Could there be bias in the data which the study (a) does not recognise or (b) is not able to correct for?

- Are there any limitations of the data-gathering methods or of the data which the study does not describe, or does not take into account?

being assessed. In some comparative research it is important that a data-gathering method is sensitive enough to correctly identify an event in different areas or has sufficient specificity to correctly identify that the event does not occur.

Here we are referring to the sensitivity and specificity of a data-gathering method, but note that specificity is also a feature of a health screening technique. It is an evaluation criterion which we would use in a comparison of different screening methods.

Chapter 6 considers the procedures used by different data-gathering methods to maximise reliability and validity.

# 5 Validity of the analysis

The fifth set of criteria for deciding whether a study makes a true comparison refers to whether the research analysed the data using methods thought to be suitable for the type of data and the purpose of the research. Different methods are used for analysing qualitative data to those used for quantitative data, and these are discussed in more detail at the end of Chapter 6. Experimental studies that have been well designed and constructed may fall down at the later stages of data analysis (e.g. 'statistical conclusion invalidity'; Cook & Campell, 1979). We also need to note that data analysis does not, of itself, prove anything, for as Black (1993) notes:

*Statistical tests only confirm that whatever was observed did or did not (probably) happen by chance alone, indicating indirectly how likely that there was a cause. Justification of the cause is a matter for the researcher.*

---

**Box 4.5: Assessing the data analysis – summary checklist**

- Does the study use analysis techniques that are normally accepted as the best to use for this type of data and question, or justify the analysis techniques which are used?

- What is the evidence that the data analysis techniques were applied correctly or incorrectly?

- Is there a clear and acceptable description of any adjustments made for possible differences in how the data were collected in different places or for different populations?

# 6 Validity of the conclusions

Conclusions refer to the empirical findings, to any explanations – both those rejected and those proposed – and any recommendations. Are the conclusions true? A necessary condition for valid conclusions are valid concepts, design, data and analysis, as noted above, but these are not sufficient in themselves. The study must show a logical link between the questions, design, data gathering and analysis, and the conclusions. If it does not, then the validity of the conclusions are 'not proven'.

All possible limitations in design and data gathering need to be stated and all possible alternative explanations properly considered before conclusions are stated. In research with hypotheses, the conclusions normally show that an hypothesis is either disproved or that there is no evidence to disprove it; be suspicious of a conclusion which states that the evidence proves a hypothesis.

If the research does show the logical links – the chain of reasoning – and if the other aspects of the research are valid, then the conclusions may be said to be valid.

---

**Box 4.6: Assessing the conclusions or recommendations – summary checklist**

If the study meets all the above criteria, then:

- Does the research show the logical links between questions, design, methods, data, analysis and conclusions?

- If explanations or interpretations are given, are there any possible alternative explanations or interpretations which are not considered?

- Is sufficient justification given for rejecting alternative explanations or interpretations?

- Are there conclusions which are not supported by the evidence, and, if so, is this stated?

- Are valid conclusions drawn from the analysis, or justifications given for recommendations?

---

## Invalid comparisons: some causes

One way to summarise the above discussion is to note some of the causes of invalid comparison. The following lists some examples from comparative studies:

INVALID 'WHOLE OBJECT' COMPARISON OR CONCEPT COMPARISON

- Institutions considered to be 'hospitals' in one place are considered to be 'nursing homes' in another place.

- No concept (e.g. one culture in the comparison does not have a concept of 'suicide').

- Concept non-equivalence (e.g. 'suicide' is defined differently in different places).

DESIGN

- Poor sampling for the purpose of the research. Non-comparable samples (e.g. populations in two areas are compared where one population has a recent high immigrant rate).

- Data gathering was carried out at different times and no allowance was made for events that could have influenced one set of data and reduced their comparability.

DATA-GATHERING METHODS

- Invalid operationalisation of the study concept(s).

- Different concept operationalisation in different places (e.g. the categories for recording are different).

- The data-gathering methods used are different in different places.

DATA QUALITY

- Researcher or data-recorder differences: differences in data recording in training.

- Differences in subject response styles in different areas (e.g. extremity scoring).

- Differences in subject familiarity with the items in a survey.

- Differences in social acceptability or desirability of response (e.g. alcohol consumption in France and south Norway).

- Different physical conditions for data gathering.

- Poor translation.

## Conclusions

- There are some principles and concepts that apply to all types of comparative health research, and which help to assess or plan a comparative study:

  - there should be a clear question or hypothesis which is significant

  - the purpose of the research should be clear (Who is the research for? What do they want or need to know? Why do they want or need to know this? Why is a comparative study necessary to discover this?)

  - the whole object comparison and the conceptual comparison made in the study should be valid

  - the operational concepts used in different places should be valid, and the data-gathering methods should be reliable in the different places they are used

  - there should be clear, logical connections between question, design, data and results, and the conclusions should be justified.

- Some criteria for assessing or planning a study are specific to the perspective used; the criteria for experimentalist studies are different to those for subjectivist studies.

- A full checklist for assessing or designing a comparative research study which uses the criteria discussed in this chapter is given in Appendixes 2 and 3.

# 5

# Eight designs for comparative health research

*Most comparative studies use one of eight types of research design. Identifying the design used in a particular study helps us to quickly make sense of the study and apply the right criteria to assess it. The ability to decide the right type of design is important, both for users to assess a study and for researchers to plan a comparative study.*

## Introduction

This chapter describes some of the more common types of research designs used in comparative health research. We look at eight designs, three of which are 'descriptive', two of which are 'epidemiological' and three of which are 'experimental'. The aim is to enable you to identify the type of design used in a study, or which you might use if you are planning one. Being able to identify which design a study uses helps you to more quickly understand the study and to see its strengths and weaknesses. It helps to see which problems threaten the validity of the study and which problems are less important.

Being able to outline the overall research design is important to researchers, both in planning and in presenting their study to others. Through the design, researchers consider and plan how their work will answer the research question. The chapter finishes with guidance on how to describe and summarise a comparative research study, in part by describing the design. It gives a checklist of questions for summarising and assessing the design used in a study.

The eight different types of design are:

'Descriptive comparisons'

1 survey

2 case study

3 audit

'Epidemiological designs'

4 retrospective case control

5 cohort

'Experimental designs'

6 outcome

7 prospective experimental

8 'full experimental' randomised controlled trial.

The chapter uses a standard format to describe each: examples of studies using the design, the type of phenomena compared, the purpose of the design and finally comments about the design. The following assumes that a specific question or hypothesis has been defined, and that this determines which design to use.

# Descriptive comparisons

## I Survey or statistical comparison

EXAMPLES

- A comparative survey of the alcohol consumption reported by a sample of people replying to a postal questionnaire in Denmark and Norway.

- Comparing the prevalence of a disease in two populations.

- Comparing the number of hospital beds in two or more areas.

PHENOMENA COMPARED

- The prevalence (at one time) or incidence (over a period) of a specified item such as a health state, or behaviour, or a characteristic of a person, population or organisation.

PURPOSE

- To find out whether, or how much, a phenomenon occurs in two or more places at one time.

COMMENTS

Note that 'cross-sectional study' is a term used for a study of *one* population to discover the prevalence or incidence of a disease, a behaviour or some other characteristic. Such studies aim to find the number of 'cases' and 'non-cases' in the population. A 'comparative cross-sectional study' is a study of two or more populations to discover the prevalence or incidence of the characteristic in each population. For example, a study of how many people in a rural part of Finland have diabetes compared to the number in a rural part of Sweden.

# 2 Case-study comparison

EXAMPLES

- Comparison of two hospitals in different places at one time, or over a similar time period.
- Comparison of the experience of six hospitals which introduced quality programmes.
- Comparison of a small number of individuals in different countries who live for 10 years after being diagnosed with terminal cancer.

PHENOMENA COMPARED

- A few 'cases', which may be people, organisations or health systems, and the context surrounding the case.

PURPOSE

- To describe two or more cases at one time and the context surrounding the cases, in order to discover similarities and differences, describe changes and explore the influence of the environment on the case or understand the case in its natural context.

COMMENTS

Sometimes some or all the cases are subjected to a particular intervention, for example a new method of financing is introduced to hospitals. The case comparisons may be of how these hospitals responded, or of how they responded compared to those which did not get the new system. Although this involves an intervention, such a study is not an 'experimental study' because neither the intervention nor the context are controlled; the aim of the case study is to give rich description of a few cases in a context.

*The distinguishing characteristic of the case study is that it attempts to examine: a) a contemporary phenomenon in its real-life context, especially when, b) the boundaries between context and phenomenon are not clearly evident.* (Yin, 1981)

*Conventionally, case study analysis has been used for hypothesis generation, and quasi-experimental methods for hypothesis testing ... At its best, the comparative case study method may produce powerful information as: 'two cases may appear very similar, yet experience different outcomes'. Here the goal is to identify the difference that is responsible for contradictory outcomes in at least relatively similar circumstances.* (Pettigrew *et al.*, 1992)

Case study comparisons often aim to produce generalisations from comparing a few individual cases, using the method of induction. In contrast, many survey or statistical comparisons aggregate data to describe an abstract feature of different groups. This latter design is more favoured in comparative health research because it is assumed to produce more valid generalisations. However, it is a mistake to assume that data from comparing a few cases is less generalisable than group data. Well-designed comparative case studies can produce more valid generalisations about individual cases than survey group data comparisons.

Note also that a research study could compare published case studies and their results by carrying out a meta-analysis of these studies.

# 3 Audit comparisons

EXAMPLES

- A comparison of the performance of four surgical departments in different areas against specified standards and protocols.
- The results achieved by three hospitals in relation to their assessment against the Swedish Quality Award criteria.

- A comparison of the experience of hospitals which were assessed using the Swedish Quality Award approach and those assessed using the Swedish SPRI Organisational Audit approach (a comparison of two different auditing methods).

PHENOMENA COMPARED

- The performance of people or organisations in relation to established standards or procedures (the 'audit criteria'). Their performance on these 'audit criteria' are then compared.
- The experience of people who used or were subjected to one or more auditing method.

PURPOSES

- To compare the performance of two or more people or organisations against a set of established criteria, for monitoring purposes or to decide how to improve performance.
- To discover how people respond to or experience one or more auditing methods.

COMMENTS

Comparative audits are increasingly used in applied health research and in routine monitoring, and are an important evaluation design (Øvretveit, 1998). They depend on a set of standards or procedures which are agreed and explicit, and which can be used to compare different services or people against this set. The value of an audit design for comparison depends on the set of standards being appropriate to the different people or services to which they are applied.

Studies using any of the above three 'descriptive designs' depend on theory and concepts that guide the descriptions and define the phenomena which are to be compared. In some, the research is carried out inductively, discovering similarities and differences as the research proceeds (e.g. in some case studies). In others, theory is used to construct a framework before the data gathering, or a hypothesis is defined which is tested in the comparison. However, none of these descriptive designs involve a planned and controlled intervention, and it is this which distinguishes these studies from 'experimental' studies.

# Epidemiological comparisons

## 4 Retrospective comparative case control

EXAMPLE

- A study of people with leukaemia in one area compared to people in another area who do not have leukaemia, but who are in all respects similar apart from being resident in the area for longer than 10 years.

PHENOMENA COMPARED

- People or organisations with a characteristic in one area ('cases') are compared with people or organisations without the characteristic in another area, but who are in all other respects similar ('controls').

PURPOSE

- To discover by 'looking backwards' why people or organisations in one area have a characteristic which people or organisations in another area do not have, where statistical analysis and control of confounding variables is possible.

- More specifically: to test one or more hypotheses about the relation between a dependent variable (characteristic) and independent variables (factors in the context).

COMMENTS

If a descriptive comparison has previously discovered a high prevalence of disease in one area, it may then be worthwhile to carry out a retrospective comparative case–control study. The aim would be to discover factors in the past which may be associated with the presence or absence of the disease in the present; there is sufficient knowledge to justify a study and to define one or more testable hypotheses.

Case–control studies are normally termed 'observations' rather than experimental studies because they do not make a deliberate intervention to the people or organisations which are studied. Rather, the people or organisations are studied in a way which aims to test whether their characteristics (dependent variable) are associated with, or even caused by, a hypothesised 'intervention(s)' in the past (i.e. independent variable(s)).

# 5 Cohort comparison

EXAMPLES

- A longitudinal study of the health of government employees in Iceland, Denmark, Norway, Sweden and Finland.

- A study of the change in lifestyle of people in urban and rural areas who were diagnosed with cancer at a similar time.

PHENOMENA COMPARED

- The health, behaviour or characteristics of two or more groups of people ('cohorts') over a period of time into the future.

PURPOSE

- To discover what happens to the people in the future, in respect of their disease or some other characteristic, by studying the two or more groups over a period of time.

COMMENTS

Cohort studies may be exploratory, but a good design will always have a specific hypothesis to test when following the people in the cohort. The cohort design differs from an experimental design in that there are no deliberate interventions made by the researchers. However, some cohort studies can involve a control group without the specified characteristics, but who are 'matched' so that they are in all respects the same.

Some researchers confusingly use 'cohort' also to describe studies which examine the past experience of one or more groups (retrospective):

*A cohort study can be either retrospective, for example reviewing all cases of three types of cancer in seven Californian hospitals between 1980 and 1982, or prospective, that is identifying a group of healthy people or patients and following them from one point in time to another.* (Gray, 1997)

The summary in this chapter follows convention in using 'cohort' only for prospective studies, as described by Crombie (1996):

*The defining characteristic of cohort studies is the element of time: in cohort studies time flows forwards. A set of individuals is identified at one point of time, and followed up to a later time to ascertain what has happened. The direction of time is always forward. Studies in which individuals are selected at one point and traced backwards to see how they were at some time previously are not cohort studies.*

# Experimental comparisons

## 6 Comparison of outcome (or 'before and after') experiments

EXAMPLES

- The effects on patient behaviour and health of a standardised stop-smoking intervention carried out by primary health care physicians in Denmark and Sweden.

- The effects on health employee attitudes and behaviour of quality training programmes given in six different hospitals.

PHENOMENA COMPARED

- The effect on people which is thought to be attributable to an intervention in one place compared to the effect of the same or a similar intervention on another group of people in one or more other places.

PURPOSE

- To discover whether an intervention has the same effect on people in two or more different places.

- To discover the effects of similar interventions on different people in different places.

COMMENTS

This design compares one group of people who get an intervention in one place with (an)other group(s) who get the same or a similar intervention in another place. It compares the before and after difference in one group with the before and after difference of one or more groups elsewhere. A clear hypothesis is an essential prerequisite.

It is the first of the three experimental designs described here, so called because the design involves planning an intervention and then studying what happens as if it were an experiment. Unlike the two other experimental designs, this simple before–after design does not control for factors other than the intervention which could explain the outcome, or the differences between different outcomes in different places.

# 7 Prospective experimental comparative case control

EXAMPLES

- A study is planned to examine the results and experience of primary health care centres which introduce alternative therapists with centres which do not, but which are similar in other respects.

- Patient outcomes after undergoing day surgery in a new unit are compared with patient outcomes in another centre without new day surgery methods.

PHENOMENA COMPARED

- The effect on 'cases' (people or organisations) of an intervention compared to 'controls' which do not get the intervention.

PURPOSE

- To discover the effects of a planned intervention by comparing the effects of the intervention on people or organisations in one place compared to the effects on people or organisations in another place.

COMMENTS

The best way to test an idea in an experiment is to plan and then make the experiment prospectively. A 'prospective case control' is planned and an intervention is made to the experimental group in one place, while no intervention is made to the control group in the other place.

Note that this is a different design from the 'prospective cohort' study, which does not involve an intervention. It is also different from a 'case study comparison', where an intervention might be made, but if it is, the intervention is not controlled – the aim of this design is to study the case in its context.

# 8 Randomised controlled trial

EXAMPLES

- People with a rare disease are selected and then randomly allocated to a new surgical technique in one place and to a conventional treatment in another place.

- Organisations in different areas are selected to take part in a study and are randomly allocated to the experimental group, which receives training in how to improve continuity of care for patients, and a control group, which does not receive training but which is surveyed and treated in the same way in all other respects.

- The results of three drug RCTs which follow the same protocols are compared in a meta-analysis.

PHENOMENA COMPARED

- The effect on people or organisations of an experimental intervention compared to the effect on those not receiving the intervention. Or the results of two or more published RCTs are compared in a meta-analysis.

PURPOSE

- To discover whether the effects are due to the intervention, by maximising the control over all factors which might give alternative explanations for any effects discovered.

COMMENTS

Experimental designs try to control through a pre-study planning of all possible influences or explanations other than the planned intervention. The aim is to discover if there is any effect that is greater than chance which can then be attributed to the intervention rather than to other influences. Normally, experimental designs aim to test both experimental groups and control groups in the same as near-laboratory conditions as possible, in order to increase control over confounders and standardise the intervention.

The advantage of allocating subjects randomly to the intervention group and to the control group is that if enough subjects are used we can rule out inherent characteristics of the subjects as one explanation for any differences between the two groups – it allows greater control than 'matching' subjects.

One variant of this design is where the results from one case control experiment in one country are compared to the results in another country. For example, one group of researchers carry out a trial of a new drug in one country and their results are compared with those of researchers using the same design and research protocols in another country (e.g. Drummond *et al.*, 1992). Doing so can reveal other factors that may influence results which are not revealed in a single country trial.

# Summarising and assessing a design

What is the best way to assess a design for a comparative study? This final part of the chapter shows ways to summarise the main features of a design and how to assess a design. We assume here that a research question or hypothesis has been defined (Chapter 4 gives guidance on how to do this). The design is constructed to answer the research question. If there is no clear question or hypothesis, then we cannot decide or assess a design. This is true even for exploratory and descriptive comparative studies.

## Could the design answer the research question or test the hypothesis?

There are two main questions for assessing a design, which are also relevant for researchers planning a study. First, 'Is a design of this type capable in principle of answering the research question?' (the potential of the design to answer the question). Second, 'Could a design of this type be properly completed with the resources available?' (the practical feasibility).

When summarising a study in order to answer these questions, we concentrate on the following features: the general type of comparison made, the actual items compared, the sampling used for data gathering, the type of data-gathering methods or measures used, and the timing of data gathering. The quickest and most effective way to summarise a design is to draw it using the diagram like Figure 3.1, with notes on the diagram to show the timing and methods of data gathering.

## General and specific comparisons

The first step in summarising a design is to state the general type of comparison which a study makes (i.e. the type of 'whole objects' compared). Is the study comparing populations (e.g. diseases or death rates in different populations) or different health organisations, health systems or health policies, or the same policy applied in different places? What is the general definition used to describe the thing being compared?

The general type of comparison is different from the actual comparisons made by the study, which is the second thing a summary should state. Which particular populations, organisations or other actual 'whole objects' were compared in the study, and which data were gathered? If it was a comparative study of mortality, which specific populations were compared and how were these selected? (This is different from sampling a sub-population for data gathering, which is discussed below.) If it was a comparative study of how a health policy was implemented, which actual implementation processes were considered? If hospitals are compared, which ones, why were these selected and is this a valid selection in relation to the question?

When considering the comparison made there is usually a third aspect of design: the actual sample that was chosen for data gathering. Some comparative epidemiological studies do not use samples but compare rates in whole populations. However, most studies select a sample from a population which is to be compared. A number of populations are selected for comparison and data is then collected about a sub-sample (from each area) that is thought to be representative of each of the populations. Both the general and the specific comparisons should follow from the research question or hypothesis and be justified in relation to it.

## Selection and sampling

Design questions of selection and sampling arise in all types of comparative research. In comparisons of health organisations the selection question that arises is which specific organisations to study for the purposes of the comparison. Some studies deliberately choose a particular service or groups of services because they exemplify a feature that is of interest (e.g. are considered successful or innovative). This is 'purposive' or 'systematic selection' for case studies. Such studies then have to decide the basis for sampling people or other data units within the organisation for data gathering.

We can rarely get data from every member of a 'population' (as in a census), such as all the people who received a treatment, or who work in a service, or who live in an area and are the target of a health policy. If we use a sample, we need to know how representative this sample is of a larger population. Care is needed in selecting a sample before gathering data so that generalisations and valid inferences can be made later.

There are a number of sophisticated methods for sample design and statistical analysis. Generally the options are random sampling (each person has a random chance of being selected, as in 'randomised trials'), cluster sampling (selecting by random a cluster from within a selected sample of areas or organisations) or quota sampling which selects 'quotas' of the population which represent one or a few features of the larger population (e.g. a certain number of the same age and sex as the larger population). A minimum total number in a sample is also important for some statistical tests of significance.

A short summary of sampling in health care is given in Sapsford and Abbott (1992, pp. 89–93), St Leger *et al.* (1992, pp. 164–9), and Edwards and Talbot (1994, pp. 33–4). A related issue which is important to validity is response rate or ratio. Few studies are able to gather usable data from all the people in the sample, and it is important to know the actual number sampled and how this varies from the total sample so as to be able to judge if the data are biased. The response rate or ratio is the actual number of people for whom data were recorded in relation to the total number in the sample (e.g. completed questionnaires are received from 67% of the people who were sent a questionnaire). McConway (1994, pp. 58–61) gives a

---

**Box 5.1: A checklist for summarising, assessing or planning a design**

1 Is the research question clearly defined and answerable, or the hypothesis testable?

2 Is there a clear and justified link between the question and the design?

3 What is the general type of comparison made?

4 Which actual comparisons are made?

5 How were people (or other 'data units') sampled for data gathering, if sampling was used?

6 Which data-gathering methods or measures were used?

7 At which times were data gathered (how often and over which periods)?

8 Which methods were used to analyse the data?

9 Were all aspects of context or confounding variables properly considered?

simple discussion of the issues involved, as do St Leger *et al.* (1992, pp. 167–9).

Note that 'theoretical sampling' is a specific technique for qualitative analysis. This technique is used during or after data collection within qualitative research and grounded theory approaches; it is a very different method to the 'subject sampling' noted above. Glaser and Strauss (1968) use the term to describe how the researcher reflects on data and develops concepts and hypotheses out of the data, then tests these ideas against the data or in further data collection.

## Conclusions

- A summary of the design of a comparative research study helps us to understand it, to assess it, to plan a study and to present it to other people.

- A study should be designed to answer the research question or to test the hypothesis. No question or hypothesis, no design. Poorly formulated research problem statements make it difficult to decide the best design or to assess a design.

- Designs for 'descriptive comparisons' include survey, case study and audit.

- Epidemiological comparisons often use either a retrospective case control design or a prospective cohort design.

- Experimental designs include comparisons of before and after experiments in different places, prospective experimental and 'full experimental' randomised controlled trials.

- Design involves deciding which whole objects to compare, and which sample for data gathering would allow a valid answer to the research question and generalisation of the findings.

- A summary of the design notes the general and the actual comparisons made, the data-gathering or measurement methods, when and how often the data were gathered and how they were analysed, as well as how the context was considered. A diagram is a good way to represent a design (*see* Figure 3.1 and Øvretveit, 1998).

# 6

# Data-gathering and analysis methods for comparative research

*Health researchers need to be broad-minded about methods and knowledgeable about a number of ways to gather data. Users of research need to understand how the data were produced and analysed in order to judge the validity of the conclusions. This chapter gives an introduction to the different methods for gathering data used in comparative health research.*

## Introduction

At the centre of a comparative research study is the work of collecting, recording and analysing data. Researchers tend to have a preference for particular methods, in part because these methods are suited to the subject and type of questions studied in their discipline. Yet there are many different methods that a health services researcher can use, even if they are working within traditional disciplinary boundaries. One example is the greater use being made by experimental medical researchers of interviews with patients to gather data about the patients' perceptions of outcomes, as well as using the more traditional objective measures of physiological and functional outcome. Health researchers making comparisons are even more likely to use a variety of methods. This is especially so if they are examining the context of the items they are comparing, where they often need to gain data about lifestyle, or social, economic and political factors.

This book considers research that examines many different subjects: disease, individuals' perceptions of health, organisations and policy processes, to name but a few. Consequently we need to consider many different types of data-gathering methods. There are choices to make about which methods to use and these choices depend on the nature of the item studied and on the purposes and questions of the study.

As more data about health and health services become more easily accessible, with much of the data presented in an already comparable form, the dangers of misuse and misinterpretation increase. There is an increasing temptation to let the available data, databases and comparisons shape the research question. One of the themes of this book is the importance of clarifying the research questions or hypotheses at an early stage, and to be certain which data are needed, before then considering which method is best for collecting these data. The choice of method should come last. Compromises can then be made about the method and how it is applied, knowing the ideal from which one is diverging and therefore the weaknesses of the data collected. A final point is the importance of scrupulous honesty and detail in describing the data-gathering methods and of the limitations of the data. This allows others to judge the validity of your conclusions and the implications.

This chapter gives an introduction to five categories of methods: using already collected data (such as government statistics); observation; interviewing; questionnaires and surveying; and specific measurement methods. For each category, different methods are described, and the general strengths and weaknesses of the methods for gathering data in two or more places are then considered. The latter involves a discussion of issues of conceptual validity and practical problems of administering the method in different settings, which were considered in Chapter 4. The aim is to give an overview of the range of methods and to highlight issues to consider in data gathering in comparative research.

## Data collection in the context of a research perspective

'Data gathering' describes a part of the research process where the researcher identifies sources of data, gets access to these sources and collects those data which are needed. The term 'data gathering' describes a range of methods within the following categories:

- *Already collected data*: data collected for other purposes, by a service, government departments, other researchers, opinion polls and other people (e.g. journalists) ('secondary data'), as well as diary records, minutes of meetings, patient case records, legal documents, etc. (sometimes called 'primary sources').

- *Observation*: unobtrusive, participant or self-observation.

- *Interviews*: structured (e.g. questions), semi-structured, open or guided by a critical incident or vignette stimulus. Focus group interviews.

- *Questionnaire or survey*: small- or large-scale survey, with or without rating scales.

- *Measurement methods*: biophysical, subjective response or a pre-formulated measurement instrument, such as disease-specific or quality of life composite measures.

The chapter uses the term 'data gathering' because it does not imply that some methods are any more 'valid' than others, or a hierarchy of methods, or that some data are 'hard' or 'soft'. The chapter does assume that some methods are better than others for certain purposes and subjects, and that some give more valid knowledge than others about particular phenomena.

# What are facts or data? – the perspective of this book

The terms 'data gathering' or 'collection' imply both an empiricist and positivist view: that facts 'lie around' waiting to be collected by a 'scientific vacuum cleaner'. This is not the view taken by this book, which does not see facts as existing independently of an observer, but neither does it regard facts as being entirely constructed by the mind of the observer – data 'production' or 'creation' would also be slightly misleading terms.

The view taken here is that facts are created in a relationship between the observer and the observed (interaction), and through relationships between observers who agree what is to be counted a fact or how to gather factual information (intersubjective agreement about procedures). Facts and evidence do not exist before or without the method for 'gathering' or 'creating' them or without pre-observational categories. The approach taken here emphasises that what is to be accepted as a fact or as evidence depends on the categories brought to bear by the researcher in gathering data. Whether data are 'valid evidence' also depends on the method being used in the right way, using techniques to maximise validity and reliability.

Before discussing each category of methods, there are a few final intro-ductory points to be made about how the methods are used within the overall research perspective used for a particular study:

1 The way a data-gathering method is used depends on the perspective of the research (*see* Chapters 1 and 3). An experimentalist approach will use data collection to test hypotheses, and will have carefully pre-defined concepts and measures. A subjectivist or phenomenological study will work more inductively, building up concepts and hypotheses from the

data. Both perspectives may use interviewing or observation, but will be using these data-gathering methods in different ways.

2 Some methods are termed 'quantitative' because they assign numbers to an aspect of a person, organisation or event. 'Qualitative data-gathering methods', on the other hand, are methods for recording and understanding people's experiences and the meanings which they give to events, and their behaviour in natural settings. For simplicity, the chapter follows the traditional terminology of describing methods as 'qualitative' or 'quantitative', even though these terms should be applied to data not to the methods. Some methods, such as interviewing, can be used to gather data in a qualitative or quantitative form.

3 Qualitative data are often gathered as part of an inductive approach, which seeks to build up categories of meaning from the data, usually out of people's reported experiences and perceptions, or from observations of their behaviour. In this way the researcher defines categories after and sometimes during data collection, rather than before. In some comparative research this may involve researchers in different sites co-operating closely at different times in order to compare the concepts that are emerging from their interviews. 'Qualitative research' is research which only uses qualitative methods. For some purposes this gives more valid data than quantitative methods, but these data may be less reliable.

4 Strictly speaking, we can only assess the suitability of a data-gathering method in relation to the particular questions and hypotheses of a study. We can only assess the quality of data in relation to the research question and purpose of the research. Thus there is no such thing as the 'general validity' of a measure or data-gathering method, only validity in relation to a particular purpose or concept. Validity refers to how a concept stated in the research question or hypothesis is operationalised, or the validity of a method for building up concepts from subjects' perceptions in order to answer a particular research question.

## Using existing data sources

*Do not collect data which someone else has already collected, if you can use their data for your purposes. But always assume such data are unreliable, not valid or comparable, unless you can prove otherwise. These are the two general rules.*

'Existing data' are data already collected for purposes other than the research, and include government statistics, hospital or primary care centre administrative data and patient records. Here we will consider the methods commonly used to collect these data and the methods that comparative health researchers can use to find, abstract and analyse these data.

Before using already collected data be careful to check how it was collected and whether you can use it for the research you are carrying out. The main problems are finding out if any data which you might be able to use already exists, and then finding out the details of how the data were collected and recorded (the methods used by others). We need to know which methods were used in order to judge the validity and reliability of the data and to decide if we can use the data for our purposes.

# Step 1: Finding and accessing data sources

The first step is to identify possible sources of already collected data ('secondary sources'). This step depends on being clear which types of data are required to answer the research question. What are we comparing (concept and operational definition)? What do we need to know about context, if anything? Which data do we need about which aspects of context? Over which timescale are the data required? Answers to these questions help to suggest possible sources of existing data.

There are different methods for searching for sources. We can get a published hard copy of reported data and search manually using the index and contents, or we can carry out an electronic search using a computer disk or Internet search method (Gray, 1997). The more commonly used databases are noted in Appendixes 2 and 3.

For data for comparisons within one country we can search within national government statistics to see if the data are reported there. Most national governments collect data about populations and about public services for a variety of purposes. For example, since 1749 data has been collected nationally in Sweden on annual births and deaths, and since 1930 a Census of Population and Housing has provided a range of detailed data every 10 years, and every 5 years since 1960. Similar sources exist within Nordic countries including national disease registers (e.g. cancer registers) and other registers, some of which are run by medical specialties (Garpenby & Carlsson, 1994). There are also comparative databases issued by the Nordic Council (NCM, 1995; NOMESCO, 1996).

In the UK, a 10-year national population census has been carried out since 1801 (apart from 1941), and details of a 1% sample of this census are also collected. St Leger *et al.* (1992) describe other sources of data in the UK, including population 'deprivation' measures, national interview surveys such as the General Household Survey, health statistics such as births and deaths, and occupational mortality and morbidity indicators.

*The steady expansion and improving quality of the OECD health database files simplifies international comparative health studies and makes them more attractive to use.* (Kroneman & van der Zee, 1997)

If we are undertaking a Nordic, European or wider international comparison we can search a number of databases to see if the data we require are reported. Most are now on CD ROM, allowing computer searches and data manipulation. Nordic databases reporting morbidity and mortality, as well as many other data, include NOMESCO (1996) and NCM (1995), and commonly used European databases include WHO (1992), Eurostat (1992) and, for OECD countries, OECD (1990, 1993a,b).

Other methods for finding sources, mostly for within-country comparisons, include asking service providers or clerical staff if there are records, statistics and other sources which might give the data needed for the research. The researcher can also look at public or private indexes or registers of documents held by institutions. For identifying data published in research reports and journals there are a variety of databases, such as MEDLINE, Social Science Citations Indexes and those for health management and policy, such as the Leeds University UK 'HELMIS' database. The quickest way to search is using an electronic database such as MEDLINE, which is available on CD ROM or over the Internet. Researchers can access some databases through the Internet and search directly, but usually only if they or their institution subscribes to the database and they can get a password for the search; charges are often by subscription and then by amount of time of use. Books and papers on 'evidence-based healthcare' describe different methods to search for publications (e.g. Gray, 1997).

Statistics about services include data about inputs and processes such as bed numbers, admissions, staffing and sometimes data about outcomes. Health service activity and performance data include: numbers referred, numbers using the service, numbers discharged, age and sex and other patient characteristics, types of needs/diagnoses, types and numbers of treatments provided, throughput, bed utilisation, average length of treatment, waiting lists, waiting times, unit costs, staffing numbers/grades, absenteeism, sickness and turnover. Some countries also have national or local statistics on number of patients for the major Diagnostic Related Groups (DRGs).

It is possible that individual patient case records might contain the data required, but there are likely to be great variations in how data are recorded and problems in gaining access. These sources are already used for some types of research, such as some quality assurance procedures or audit. Medical and other types of audit reports are also useful data sources for some research (e.g. NCEPOD, 1987, 1989, 1993).

An important set of issues to consider in deciding whether to use existing data concerns confidentiality, access and ethics. These issues do not arise with published sources (although permission to reproduce might), but confidentiality issues do arise if one is abstracting from some administrative patient databases and from primary sources such as patient records. There are usually strict rules to ensure patient confidentiality, which researchers will need to understand and respect. The researcher may be allowed access to the data, but can they publish the data, or what changes would be required to allow publication? Who owns data that is not already public?

*International comparisons are only as good as the basic underlying data upon which they are based.* (Shieber & Poullier, 1989)

## Step 2: Assessing data sources

*The wisest policy is conservatism: when using 'comparable datasets' the researcher should expect that the data are not comparable until they have proven otherwise by finding out the details of data collection and assessing validity and reliability.*

The second step in this method of data gathering is to assess the already collected data for the purposes of the research. Common problems in using published international and national comparisons of raw statistics are that the data-gathering methods are not described, or there are countries or data missing from the full set. The most usual is that there are differences in classification or definition between countries, which may not be clear in the published tables or background discussions.

For example, information about services for older people are often classified differently, in part because much care for the elderly lies on the boundary between health and social services and can be the responsibility of different agencies in different countries. A problem in compiling the 1989 OECD Health Data File was that Sweden classified 'nursing' beds as part of 'inpatient medical care', while in Denmark, 'inpatient medical care beds' data did not include 'residential' beds, which were provided under the Social Affairs Ministry. This problem also applies to in-country time comparisons: after 1992, Swedish national health expenditure statistics no longer include expenditure for residential care for older people, so that comparisons across time are difficult.

Other examples are the category 'licensed health professionals', which includes chiropractors in some countries and not in others, and 'pharmaceutical consumption', which in some countries does not include hospitals, and where it does, it may not include medicines given in outpatient clinics. Similarly, physicians in some countries are allowed to dispense medicine (e.g. in urban Japan) and units of medicine consumed may not include their figures. In France, one prescription form may include more than three items, whereas in most other countries 'prescription' refers to a single item. In the USA, hospital expenditure typically does not include physicians, who are hospital-salaried employees in many European countries, and the word physician itself means doctor in the USA and specialist in internal medicine in the UK.

Doctors in different countries make different diagnoses of the same symptoms. For example, Fletcher *et al.* (1964) found that the high rate of 'chronic bronchitis' in England compared with the USA was in part due to doctors in the USA classifying patients with the same symptoms as suffering from 'emphysema'. Other differences in diagnosis in five European countries were noted by O'Brien (1984). Cultural differences in diagnosis are even greater in psychiatry, for example in the diagnosis of schizophrenia in France compared with the UK (Van Os *et al.*, 1993).

Although much work has been put into standardising concepts – especially for diseases – and the more recent Nordic, European and WHO datasets are much better for comparative purposes, there will always be problems. When using 'comparable datasets' the researcher should be cautious and expect that the data are not comparable until they have proven otherwise by finding out the details of data collection and assessing validity and reliability.

Assessing already collected data means applying the same tests to these data as would be applied to data gathered using a direct method such as an interview or questionnaire. The tests include validity, reliability, sampling and tests of appropriate analysis if the data are already presented as composite measures. Some of these tests were discussed in Chapter 4 when looking at validity, and Appendix 3 gives a checklist for assessing data. We consider these tests when we look at each of these methods in more detail below.

The general validity and reliability of Swedish sources is discussed in Rosen (1987), and of medical registers in Garpenby and Carlsson (1994). Some specific secondary sources are discussed in Gissler *et al.* (1995) (data quality after restructuring the Finnish 'medical birth registry'). The poor quality of the small amount of data on inpatient maternity care in the

UK is discussed in Middle and MacFarlane (1995). A good discussion of the international data comparability, especially expenditure data, is given in the 1989 supplement to the 'Health Care Financing Review' (Poullier, 1989).

# Step 3: Analysing data

The third step is to abstract from the data sources those data which are needed for the research, and to analyse these abstracted data. Often the researcher will be using already collected quantitative data and they will analyse it using statistical and other methods, depending on their assessment in step 2. The data may be qualitative, as, for example, in descriptions in case records or minutes or agenda of meetings. If so, the researcher uses coding or other methods of abstraction and data analysis for qualitative data, always bearing in mind that the text was recorded for purposes other than the research.

Although one has to know the limitations of the data, in my experience the detective work to discover already collected data is well worth the effort, especially if these data pass the second step described above. Sometimes finding out that there are no collected or recorded data, or that the data are incomplete or not comparable is itself an important finding.

More details about using existing data to compare health care reforms are given by Kroneman and van der Zee (1997), and the problems and solutions they examine are also relevant for comparisons of policies and interventions to health care organisations. They propose a research process to 'reconstruct the reform' by using 'secondary sources' such as OECD reports as a starting point. These data are used, together with 'primary sources' such as legal texts, to write a document summarising the reform or policy, which is then discussed with a variety of in-country experts representing different sectors. They also propose producing a 'reform implementation index' for each country to show the extent of implementation in the years before and after the formal reform. Further general discussions of different databases and their use and limitations for comparative research can be found in Poullier (1989), OECD (1990) and Schaapveld et al. (1995).

# Observation

Observation methods are used to collect data about the behaviour of people. These may be patients, or people who are providing a treatment or service or implementing a policy, or others such as carers, voluntary workers or politicians. 'Behaviour' is what people do and say. 'Observation' has also been used to describe a researcher analysing documents.

Different observation methods are frequently used in health service research, but less so in comparative studies. This is because it is more difficult in comparative research to ensure that different observers use observational methods in a reliable way, and to ensure the validity of the observation methods, especially if different observers from different countries are gathering the data. The following describes common observational methods and their strengths and weaknesses.

Observation can be carried out by using a pre-structured, coded observation form, or by 'open' observation, and each of these methods may be used by an independent observer or a participant observer. One particularly useful method for gaining data about a service process is to observe and record what happens to a patient as the researcher follows them in their 'journey' from admission to discharge or beyond (a 'Tracer-patient pathway study'; Øvretveit, 1994c). This can be combined with interviewing the patient to gather their perceptions at different stages.

If used within a qualitative paradigm, 'open' observation allows researchers skilled in this method to study what people do in a natural setting and to build up a conceptualisation which reflects people's behaviour in this setting. The aim here is not to impose pre-defined categories and 'count' behaviour, as would be the approach using this method within an experimental paradigm, but to 'suspend' the observer's categories and carefully record what is observed in 'field notes' during or shortly after. The aim is to observe and record as 'faithfully' and 'factually' as possible, for example by recording the words used rather than summaries. This can mean video or audio recording, although this can influence people's actions even more than the presence of the observer. Such methods have uses in comparative studies which seek to understand how people in different countries or cultures interpret or react to experiences or situations, for example by observing the behaviour of nurses in different countries when under stress or high work pressures.

'Participant observation' is a method that reduces the influence of the observer on people's behaviour, but requires the 'participant observer' to take part in everyday life for some time, sometimes without disclosing their role as an observer. This increases validity but still leaves a question as to whether a similarly trained observer would see and record the same things. There are also ethical problems with the participant observer role. For example, some view it as deliberate deception and betraying the trust of patients and health care workers.

## Strengths and weaknesses for comparative health research

The strengths of observation methods are that they give direct evidence of observed outcomes and processes, rather than reported accounts. Data from observation can be used to develop theories about how the context affects behaviour and why people react as they do. Observation also gives real examples which capture the flavour of the setting. But while there are some uses for this method, there are four 'threats' to validity which make it a less attractive method for those who are not trained anthropologists or sociologists. There are problems in ensuring the reliability of observations so that valid comparisons can be made. Second, the effect of the observer on what people would otherwise do is likely to be greater if they know that the observer is a researcher who may be publishing their findings. This effect may be different in different countries or cultures. Third, pre-coded observation categories, if they are used, may ignore the different meanings of the same behaviour in different countries or cultures.

The fourth threat to validity applies to the use of this method within a qualitative paradigm where the observer does not use pre-set categories. How do we know whether the observer imposes their categories or 'distorts' what they observe? The observer has to have some categories or ways of seeing to decide what to observe and record – there is no such thing as 'open observation'. Qualitative researchers recognise these criticisms and have a number of strategies to reduce observer bias and increase validity. They emphasise that: the categories are built up inductively and stress the ideal of factual description; that records provide evidence which can be checked by others, including the participants ('participant validation'); that multiple observers are used; and that observation is one of multiple sources of data ('triangulation'; Jick, 1983).

These and other problems and details of the observational method in conventional health research are described in outline in McConway (1994, pp. 22–6, with examples from bedside medical teaching), Mays and Pope (1995, pp. 182–4) and in more detail in Sapsford and Abbott (1992, pp. 127–35). Practical general accounts are given in Edwards and Talbot (1994, pp. 76–85) and how to use pre-coded observation is described in Breakwell and Millward (1995). More detailed discussions can be found in general texts on social science methods, such as Adams and Shvaneveldt (1991). How to analyse qualitative data from observation and from interviews is a subject considered later.

# Interviewing

Interviewing gives the researcher access to people's views, their recollected experiences, feelings and their theories about causation. This method can be used to collect data in a quantitative form, where the interviewer uses pre-structured categories and questions (e.g. a pre-coded questionnaire administered in an interview). It can also be used to collect qualitative data by using open-ended questions or a set of topics for open exploration and probing by the interviewer. Here we consider interviewing as a method for collecting qualitative data, used within a qualitative paradigm.

In-depth interviewing can be semi-structured with a set of topics or unstructured, where the interviewer is led by the person's concerns and aims to discover what a person's views are and why they hold these views. This type of interviewing is a skilled task requiring the interviewer to demonstrate interest without becoming over-involved and biased, to gain trust, to appear neutral and non-judgemental to the person, and to know when and how to probe when something of general interest to the research arises. The 'therapeutic' dimension of interviewing in health care research is noted later in this section. During some research, interviewers may change their interview strategies so as to pursue topics and hypotheses that have emerged out of previous interviews.

Interviews are useful for gaining data about patients' experiences in their own terms. Interviews can find out patients' recollected experiences, for example of their situation and expectations before undergoing a treatment or a service. Interviews also allow the researcher to discover how health service personnel understood or responded to an intervention or policy. This is important data for understanding how or why some policies work or fail – the perceptions of staff and their reasons for acting in the way they do can be useful data for all types of research. A policy or change often has a meaning or symbolic importance which is not recognised by outsiders, but may be critical to the impact of an intervention – this is as true for interventions into health services as it is for health education programmes to particular groups. How people interpret change is important for understanding the effects, and interviews are the main way of gathering data about how people interpret and understand interventions. Researchers can build theories about how an intervention works or fails, either by testing their own theories in interviews or by seeking out and refining participants' theories.

Before considering the strengths and weaknesses of interview methods for comparative research, we will note one type of group interview.

## Focus group interview method

The advantage of an 'interview' with a group rather than with individuals is the ability to gain a range of views more quickly and with less resources than a series of interviews. The focus group technique is one form of group interview where the 'facilitator-interviewer' leads a group of about eight people in a discussion of a particular topic. As with interviews, there may be an agenda, or the facilitator may allow the discussion to develop with little prompting or probing, or may give example situations (e.g. 'critical incidents') or vignettes to stimulate views. If it is a group of people with similar backgrounds, then they usually feel less inhibited, but this may mean that the research will need many different focus groups to ensure that a range of views are captured.

People in a group with 'similar' people are usually less intimidated by the interviewer and may speak more openly and stimulate each other to recall different incidents and express views. However, it is often less easy in a group to probe and follow up one person's views, and there may also be a greater pressure to express views which a person thinks are acceptable to the group (group conformity).

The quality of the data depends even more than with individual interviews on the skills of the facilitator, and detailed recording is more difficult, although video or tape recording may be possible. These drawbacks make it a data-gathering method which is rarely used for comparative health research. However, it has been used in comparisons of the quality of different health services.

Summaries of focus group technique in health services can be found in Fitzpatrick and Boulton (1994, p. 108) and Kitzinger (1995, pp. 299–302). More details are given in books on the subject by Morgan (1993) (e.g. when to use focus groups and why, pp. 3–19) and Kreuger (1988). An example of focus group technique in peer-service quality research is given in Øvretveit (1988), and its use in patient satisfaction research in Øvretveit (1991).

# Strengths and weaknesses of interview methods for comparative research

Thus qualitative interviewing is a method for discovering people's experiences, the meaning of events to them, their feelings and their 'lay theories'. But, as with observation, there are drawbacks and problems of validity and reliability for comparative health research. Would a similarly trained interviewer have gathered the same data? How does one analyse pages of interview transcript and how would a research user judge whether the conclusions were really based on the interview data or whether the interviewer biased the subjects' responses? How can we ensure consistency between interviewers, especially in different countries.

To some extent interviews create data in the sense that interviewees often have not thought about the issues they are asked about. Interviewees usually do not simply report their experiences, but they create or make more explicit what they think during the interview. The skill of the interviewer is to enable the person to reflect on and develop their ideas, without introducing the interviewer's own biases. A second validity issue is that the interviewee may not recollect 'properly' or may have a selective view of the event. Golden (1992) describes work which shows that managers recollect with 'hindsight bias' and in ways which unconsciously maintain their own self-esteem – she describes methods to reduce this bias and emphasises the need to acknowledge the limitations of such data.

A third validity issue is that interviewees may be more concerned with projecting the right image and with how they appear than with representing 'the truth'. For example, men reported about 30% higher levels of morbidity when they were interviewed by women than they did when interviewed by men (Nathanson, 1978). Triangulation and corroboration can be used to increase validity, as well as probing where people give discrepant accounts, and 'respondent validation' to check emerging analyses with the people interviewed or with another group.

Investigating sensitive or 'difficult' topics with interviewing raises ethical issues. If the reader thought the description of the techniques of some types of interviewing were a bit like psychotherapy, they would be right. Techniques to put the interviewee at ease, to encourage them to 'open up', and empathising methods are recommended in some texts and are taught in training programmes for interviewers and 'qualitative researchers'. There can be problems when these techniques are used with patients or health service staff who have had a bad or traumatic experience, for example to investigate poor quality or disasters.

In these situations the researcher may be the only person to whom the patient or staff member has talked about the experience, and the researcher is using powerful techniques that will encourage them to reawaken their experience. The researcher then leaves with their data, leaving the interviewee to cope with what has been re-evoked in the interview. I have known some well-meaning 'qualitative studies' where junior researchers have been trained in these techniques but have not been able to deal with the feelings of distress they uncover; talking about an experience does not of itself cure the original trauma – more is required to help a person work through an experience after being 'opened up'. Studies need to recognise the 'therapeutic' dimension of interviewing, the ethical issues and the need for appropriate interviewer supervision.

A strength of some interview methods is that they allow the researcher to build up an understanding of the patients' and healthcare providers' experiences, meanings and feelings. They do this by understanding people in their own settings and terms. This is particularly important for gathering data about outcomes and about how interventions may work where people's feelings are an important 'mediating variable'. We noted problems of validity: the researcher may impose their own biases and categories rather than represent those of the participants; interviews often create people's views as much as they reflect views; problems in reporting the analysis and conclusions; difficulties in knowing how general the findings might be; and problems in reliability or replication.

Both observation and interviewing can be used to collect data in a quantitative or qualitative form. Later we consider methods for analysing these types of data. When choosing a data-gathering method, the researcher needs to consider how they will analyse the data and present it to users. One of the greatest weaknesses of qualitative observation and interviewing is the difficulty in analysing and presenting the data, especially to users who are unfamiliar with or skeptical of these methods.

For more details of qualitative open interviewing in health settings the reader is referred to a summary in Britten (1995, pp. 251–3) and to Sapsford and Abbott (1992, pp. 108–115), McConway (1994, pp. 27–30), who also introduces 'feminism and qualitative interviewing' in health care, and Fitzpatrick and Boulton (1994, pp. 107–8). Practical summaries are given by Edwards and Talbot (1994, pp. 86–9) and Breakwell and Millward (1995, pp. 67–73). One interesting example of the use of semi-structured interviewing is given in a study which sought older people's perceptions of care and problems (Powell *et al.*, 1994). The in-depth interview method in organisational studies is described in Ghauir *et al.* (1995, pp. 64–72). General social science methodology texts give extensive practical and theoretical discussion of the method. Kvale (1994) gives a very readable and concise discussion of 'ten standard objections to qualitative research interviews'.

## Surveying and questionnaires

Methods within this category are often used to gather data in comparative health research studies. Asking questions is one way of finding out what people think about a particular topic, and we saw above how this could be done using a semi-structured interview method. Another method is through a self-completed questionnaire, which can be mailed or completed by a person when they are in hospital, receiving care or at work. Examples of these methods include large-scale population surveys with pre-set categories and questionnaires designed to discover patients' expectations and experiences of treatment.

Questionnaires are used when researchers want to collect data about specific topics and where the topics have the same meaning and are well understood by people in different settings or social groups. Their use in comparative research thus depends on researchers understanding whether the concepts and questions in the survey are comparable between groups (see Chapter 4). Careful translation is necessary for most cross-national comparisons, although researchers need to check whether a concept applies in all populations or whether there is concept inequivalence.

Questionnaires are less expensive than interviews, which are unnecessary where simple factual data are required or where people can easily and authentically express their ideas in terms of the categories used by the researcher in the questionnaire. Questionnaires can gather qualitative data by asking people to write descriptive accounts. More often, questionnaires use one or more of a number of measurement scales which require subjects to express their views in the terms of a scale and thus provide quantitative data.

The most well-known scale is the Likert five-item scale or a Semantic Differential scale (pairs of opposites, e.g. painful–not painful, usually with a seven-point scale; see Breakwell & Millward (1995, pp. 64–6) for a simple summary). Again this can be a source of biased data, for example where people from different cultures used the extremes of rating scales in a different way (van de Vijver & Leung, 1997). The issues involved in designing and using measurement scales are discussed below. The way the questions are worded and their order are important to validity. Of particular importance in design is to look ahead to how the analysis will be performed, and with quantitative questionnaires (e.g. with rating scales) issues such as sample size need to be considered if statistically valid inferences are to be drawn from the data.

## Strengths and weaknesses

The advantages of questionnaires are that they allow people time to think and to respond anonymously. They are quick and easy to analyse (if there are few 'open questions' and they are pre-coded) and they can be given to many people at a low cost. A disadvantage is that it can be difficult to get a high response rate (over 50%) and the returned questionnaires may have a disproportionate number of people who feel particularly strongly about a topic (selective response rate), which can give misleading results if the researcher generalises the findings without noting this possibility. Other disadvantages include a proportion only being part-completed and some respondents may 'misuse' or misunderstand the categories or feel that they cannot express their view properly in the terms required. Some subjects may under- or overestimate in their replies. For example, McKinlay (1992) found that questionnaire respondents generally under-reported their alcohol consumption by about half, although he also notes that this under-reporting is even greater when respondents are interviewed.

The most well-known problem is the different responses with different question phrasing or use of terms, which adds further complications to cross-cultural studies. For example, US opinion polls found that 55% of people said they would vote for a law allowing the terminally ill to choose 'euthanasia'. This rate increased to 65% when the question was rephrased as would they support the right of the terminally ill to choose 'death with dignity' over prolonging life. 44% would allow a terminally ill person to choose a 'lethal injection' but 50% would approve a 'medical procedure'. Another UK study, when asking questions about primary care, accidentally found that over half the respondents thought primary care meant care that was more important or urgent and about 35% thought that secondary care was lower quality care. Much depends on the skill and experience of the questionnaire designer.

These and other issues are discussed in detail in general texts (e.g. Frankfort-Nachmias & Nachmias, 1992) and for research in Breakwell and Millward (1995, pp. 58–67). Questionnaire design is summarised in overviews of the method in health care in McConway (1994, pp. 57–8), Sapsford and Abbott (1992, pp. 87–100) and Edwards and Talbot (1994, pp. 99–101). McKinlay (1992, pp. 115–37) gives an excellent discussion of methods used for surveying older people. Surveys and questionnaires for organisational research are discussed in Ghauri *et al.* (1995, pp. 58–64).

There is a fine dividing line between a questionnaire survey and standard measurement instruments such as the General Health Questionnaire (Bowling, 1992). The difference is that the latter are usually constructed on the basis of an explicit conceptual model and have been extensively tested and often validated, whereas questionnaires and surveys are usually developed for the specific purpose of the research and might have little pilot testing or no validation.

## Measurement methods

*The design of controlled experimentation has been refined to a science that is within the grasp of any researcher who owns a table of random digits and recognises the difference between blind and sighted assessments. However, the measurement of outcome seems to have been abandoned at a primitive stage of development ... A superfluity of instruments exists, and too little is known about them to prefer one to another.* (Smith *et al.*, 1980)

The above critical view of outcome measures is an extreme one, and measures have advanced considerably since 1980. However, it is still true that some researchers do not choose the most appropriate outcome measure for the purpose, and this also applies to other types of measurement methods.

Measurement methods are the fifth category of data-collection methods considered here. When used as a general term, 'measurement' describes any method of data collection – questionnaires are sometimes described as measures. Here the term is used in a specific sense to mean only methods for collecting data in a numerical or 'quantified' form. More precisely, measurement is assigning numerical values to objects, events or empirical facts according to specified rules. In this sense we may measure a person's attitude by asking them to express their views in terms of a number on a rating scale (an ordinal scale), or we may measure their temperature using a thermometer (a ratio scale). We gather data not about the entity or the concept, but about the properties of a concept. This involves using indicators that are observable events which are inferred measures of concepts.

Measurement quantifies something by comparison with something else. Measures are often used in research to quantify needs and outcome, but also to quantify inputs (e.g. costing) and processes (e.g. time, the number of defined activities). Measurement is an efficient way to communicate evidence and describe things, and, if the research is well designed and conducted, can be used to discover and prove causation. In comparative health research there are three types of phenomena which are often quantified:

1 physical states, such as death and disease, or events, such as the number of hospital beds or nurses

2 activities, practices and processes, such as length of stay, financing methods and quality systems

3 perceptions and attitudes, such as employees' views about a new policy or patients' attitudes towards a new treatment.

Measures of patient outcomes used in treatment and service research include measures of physiological functioning (temperature, blood pressure, haemoglobin value, erythrocyte sedimentation rate, glucose levels, etc.), measures of physical function (e.g. activities of daily living, ability to walk, range of motion), measures of psychological functioning (e.g. response rate, cognitive abilities, depression, anxiety) and measures of social functioning (e.g. social skills, ability to participate in employment, community participation, etc.).

For comparative research we usually use numbers and a denominator, such as per 100 000 population, which are termed 'rates' (the ratio of two measures). Some comparisons are in terms of composite measures, such as a composite measure for mortality which includes infant and maternal mortality and possibly other mortality rates. Such measures are sometimes called indices or indicators, where a number of different indicators are brought together in a formula to produce one number which is then compared. In the case of a mortality composite, each mortality variable is first standardised – standardised variables are evenly distributed around zero, the average value for all the standardised variables. If the variables are given equal weighting, then the composite measure is the sum of the standard scores. Often variables are weighted differently: for example, if comparing the effects of environment on mortality the researchers might use previous research which shows the higher susceptibility of children and older people to certain environmental conditions, and give a higher weighting to child and over-65 mortality rates in the composite mortality index.

This section does not describe these different measures in detail because they are well described in general research texts such as Bowling's texts on measuring disease (Bowling, 1995) and her review of quality of life measures (Bowling, 1992), as well as in research texts such as Fink (1993), Rossi and Freeman (1993), St Leger *et al.* (1992) and Breakwell and Millward (1995).

*We value what we measure, so we must learn to measure what we value.*

## Concepts and theories underlie measures

When we measure, we or our subjects assign a number to a category – for example, age or a rating of 4 on a scale of 1 to 5. Or we read off a number from a measuring instrument such as a clock, thermometer or an EEG machine. The numbers do not pre-exist our measurement, but are created by us, our subjects or our machines, according to certain procedures. These procedures depend on a concept about the phenomenon to which a person using the procedure assigns numbers. The concept of age is one which is commonly agreed and can be measured directly – it is easy to 'operationalise' the concept in the measure of time since birth and everyone knows what it means. Note that this measure itself depends on other concepts and the measure of time. Note also that when we considered qualitative data gathering above, we faced issues of operationalisation, for example difficulties in defining a term in such a way that people understood the same thing (e.g. 'illness' or 'quality programme').

Many concepts in research are difficult to operationalise – for example 'health' – and we use indicators or proxy measures where the link between the concept and the measure is less direct than for concepts such as age.

Much health research uses numerical data from measures to describe or explain. Numbers are efficient ways for describing phenomena and allow us to see patterns when they are presented in a visual or graphical way, for example in a pie chart, histogram or scattergram. We can also describe by showing features of the numbers (which hopefully 'represent' features of the phenomenon measured), such as average and spread (e.g. standard deviation, variance, interquartile range). We can see quickly, for example, how many people who received the treatment were within different age ranges, or what proportion of the costs of a service were personnel costs. Numbers can also allow us to discover and prove causation – we consider statistical analysis below. Generally, most numerical data gathering assumes that:

- the quality or property is sufficiently important to be measured

- the method of measurement can distinguish in a useful way different amounts of the property

- the property of one item at one time that we measure can be compared to the property at another time or of another item

- the difference between, for example, '2' and '3' is equal in amount to the difference between '13' and '14' if we are using an interval or ratio scale.

---

**Box 6.1: Some common measurement terms**

*Sample*: a smaller number of a larger population

*Prevalence*: at a particular time, the number of existing cases identified or arising in a population

*Incidence*: over a period of time, the number of new cases or events identified or arising in a population

*Rate*: a ratio of two measures, such as the proportion of a population with a particular problem or characteristic, often expressed by age or by sex (e.g. cases out of 100 000). Rates require data from interval or ratio scales

*Prevalence rate* is the proportion of cases in a population at a particular time (e.g. 26 in 100 000)

*Incidence rate* is the proportion of new cases which arise over a period of time. Death or mortality rate is the proportion of a population who die – but who die during a defined time period

---

# Analysing data

*Much of the time the data are not in dispute, except where errors of observation or measurement are suspected, but it is their potential alternative interpretations which are of concern. Irrespective of the methods used, if the researcher fails to consider alternative interpretations of the findings and to discuss the merits of these alternatives, then there remain questions which serve to limit the confidence which one might have in the conclusions the author derives.* (Najman et al., 1992)

Having gathered data about items in different places, the researcher will then need to analyse the data to make a comparison, and possibly also to consider associations, causes or the influence of the context on the item. In this section we briefly note methods for analysing data in a quantitative form and for analysing qualitative data.

## Quantitative data analysis

Any data produced using measures will have errors. Some of the errors will be produced by the measurement method, and may be chance errors or systematic bias. Increasing the sample size will not reduce systematic bias in the measuring method. However, some variation is inherent in the item being studied and is not an artefact of the method. Statistical techniques are used to minimise variation and to analyse data which includes variation. Techniques for calculating statistical significance and confidence intervals help researchers and users to assess the probability of associations and to make inferences about causes.

---

**Box 6.2: Terms used in quantitative data analysis**

*Internal validity*: the validity of the conclusions in relation to the specific sample of the study. For example, in an evaluation experiment being able to show whether or not the intervention has an effect or the size of the effect

*External validity*: the ability of a study to show that the findings would also apply to similar populations, organisations or situations. For example, when an intervention is applied in another setting

*Dependent variable*: the outcome variable or end result of a treatment, service or policy which is the subject of the study (e.g. cancer mortality, patient satisfaction, resources consumed by a service) and which might be associated with or even caused by other (independent) variables. (The data analysis tests for associations between the dependent (outcome) variable and the independent variables. Establishing causation is more complex)

*Independent variable(s)*: a variable whose possible effect on the dependent variable is examined. Something which may cause the outcome and which is tested in the research. (Note: Many independent variables may be associated with a dependent variable, but only a few have a causal influence, and even fewer can be shown unambiguously to have a causal effect. A dependent variable cannot influence an independent variable: t.ex. genetic make-up can predispose to cancer, but cancer, as far as we know, cannot affect genes)

*Mediating variable(s)*: other variables which could affect the dependent variable or outcome, which the research tries to control for in design or in statistical analysis (e.g. outcome)

*Extraneous variable(s)*: variables not considered in the theory or model used in the study

*Confounding variable(s)*: any variable which influences the dependent variable or outcome but was not considered or controlled for in the study. Alternative definition: 'confounding arises when an observed association between two variables is due to the action of a third factor' (Crombie, 1996)

In many comparative studies we have two sets of numbers, for example a 'before' and an 'after' set or outcomes from two services in different places. Statistical significance testing helps to show whether or not any differences between the two sets really represents true differences in the populations from which the samples were drawn. It is based on the idea that any difference between the two sets is caused by a real difference as well as by differences arising from random and systematic error introduced by the measurement method. It involves proposing a null hypothesis – that there is no difference between the sets – and examining whether any difference shown is greater than that expected by chance. The significance level is the level of probability at which we decide to reject the null hypothesis.

*What is meant by statistically significant? It simply means that it did not occur by chance alone, there is probably some external cause … It does not prove that the variables being investigated caused the difference … It is up to the researcher to prove that the variables under consideration are the actual cause and to eliminate the possibility of any other variable(s) contributing to the results found.* (Black, 1993)

Phillips *et al.* (1994) give a useful and simple summary of the main statistical methods for analysis by distinguishing different stages of analysis. The first is to describe and summarise the data by representing each numerical value in a pie chart or bar chart, by calculating the averages (the mean, median and mode), the range (the difference between the smallest and largest value in a dataset) and the standard deviation (which is how much the data values deviate from the average). The second stage is to define the generalisability of the data by stating how much confidence we would have in finding the results from the sample in the general population. This is done by calculating the 'confidence interval'. A third 'hypothesis testing' stage involves using data to confirm or reject a hypothesis. A type I error is to reject a null hypothesis when it is in fact true: the analysis calculates the probability of having a type 1 error – called the significance level. A fourth stage is to calculate the strength of the association between two variables using chi-squared tests, calculating a correlation coefficient or carrying out a regression analysis.

Giving a short listing of these statistical methods makes them look more complicated than they are. There are now a number of texts that give simple summaries with examples. Techniques for deciding significance levels and other details of measurement, sampling and statistical analysis in health research are described in summary in St Leger *et al.* (1992, Chapter 11), Edwards and Talbot (1994, Chapter 6) and McConway (1994, Chapters 5 and 6). A simple general practical overview of 'describing and summarising data' and of drawing inferences in evaluation is given in

Breakwell and Millward (1995, pp. 80–96). Wiltkin *et al.* (1992) describe measurement of need and outcome, as does Bowling (1992, 1995). A more detailed and comprehensive text for clinicians is Gardner and Altman (1989).

## Qualitative data analysis

Perhaps the greatest problem in using qualitative data in health research – usually gathered using observation or interview methods – is analysing the data. The challenge does not stop there: there is another related problem, how to display qualitative data and to convince users and other scientists that the conclusions are justified by the data. There are two issues. First, how to use the techniques of analysis that are generally agreed by qualitative researchers to reach conclusions which other scientists using these methods would accept. Second, how to present the conclusions and analysis to those who are unfamiliar with these techniques.

Many people in health services are familiar with methods for analysing and presenting quantitative data, but not with those for qualitative data. Data analysis is one of the most difficult, time-consuming, but also creative tasks in using observation and interviewing methods within a qualitative paradigm. Analysis can be made after the data-collection phase, but within the qualitative paradigm some analysis is made during data collection. We noted this technique when describing interview methods – where an interviewer decides to follow up a subject of interest or where the interviewer formulates a hypothesis and explores it through probing and testing within the interview. A similar process of analysis is where the interviewer or team carry out an analysis after an interview and use the 'results' in subsequent interviews, these results being categories of experience or hypotheses which can be tested in other interviews. We can represent a common approach to qualitative data analysis by the following steps:

1 Interview or observation

2 Text (a write-up of the interview or field notes or transcript of a tape)

3 Code or classify (according to 'emergent' themes or patterns)

4 Further analysis (re-coding or hypothesis testing, often by returning to original text or other texts to compare views or settings for similarities and differences)

5 Conclusions/results: categories of experience or feelings of the subjects, meanings subjects give to events, explanatory models and concepts or generalisations.

Qualitative analysis is inductive, building and testing concepts in inter-action with the data or the subjects. It is also usually iterative: the analyst forms categories from the data and then returns to the data to test their generalisability.

These techniques of data analysis are complex and are not easy to describe in research reports for readers unfamiliar with the techniques, but then this is also true for methods for analysing quantitative data. However, examples from the original data give vivid illustrations and also 'ring true' with users. A comprehensive and detailed account of qualitative data analysis is given in Miles and Huberman (1984), but more simple and shorter summaries are provided in Fitzpatrick and Boulton (1994, pp. 110–11), Edwards and Talbot (1994, pp. 102–5) and Sapsford and Abbott (1995, pp. 117–25). A discussion specifically for evaluation is given in Patton (1987) and a discussion of different qualitative methods is given in Van Maanen (1983), Denzin and Lincoln (1993) and Kvale (1989).

# A technique for generating dimensions or characteristics by which to compare

A method that has uses in some studies is a technique for generating dimensions or characteristics which can then be used systematically to compare three or more different whole objects. This technique can be used in a qualitative-inductive study during or after data collection. The technique is to take three of the whole objects, and for the researcher or subjects to consider ways in which two of the objects are similar and at the same time different to a third. For example, in a comparison of three hospital quality programmes the researcher can consider ways in which two programmes are similar and thereby different to the third. The dimension might be 'top-management-initiated vs clinician-initiated', and this dimension can then be used to rate all the programmes (or descrip-tions of them) in terms of the extent to which they were top-management-initiated (rating 7) or clinician-initiated (rating 0). The technique can then be used again on another three to generate another dimension or, as Kelly terms it, 'construct'. After generating a set of dimensions and rating each object, various statistical analyses can be performed to find which objects are the most similar on a range of dimensions. Further details can be found in Kelly (1955).

# Conclusions

- Many different methods are used to gather data in the field of comparative health research, in part because of the many different types of subjects studied.

- Users of research need to have some understanding of the methods used to gather data in order to interpret the data presented in the research, to judge the validity of the conclusions and to judge the suitability of the methods proposed in a plan for a research study.

- Data for a study can be collected by using already collected data, observation, interviewing, questionnaires and surveys, and measurement methods.

- The choice of data-gathering method should follow from the research design and questions to be answered. Sometimes the reverse happens – the research design and the questions answered are decided by the data-gathering method with which the researcher is most familiar.

- Data-gathering methods are not 'scientific vacuum cleaners' for collecting facts. Facts are created through a relationship between the observer and the observed, and through relationships between observers who agree what is to be counted a fact and how to gather factual information.

- Some points to remember are:

  - define which data you need and how those data will help to answer the research question

  - consider existing data sources: which information is already collected, how accessible is it, and how valid, reliable and comparable is the information for the purposes of the research?

  - never develop a new data-collecting instrument without checking whether you could use an existing and validated instrument (the world does not need another quality of life measure)

  - if possible, combine methods to make up for each method's weaknesses

  - always estimate the time and costs and then double them (to test the method, to collect the data and to analyse the data)

  - there are no good or bad methods for gathering data, just those which are most suited to the subject and cost-effective for the purpose and questions of the research.

- When choosing a method, look ahead to how the data will be analysed and presented. In the health sector, methods for analysing quantitative data are better understood than methods for analysing qualitative data.

- It is often more difficult to judge the validity of conclusions from qualitative research using participant observation or interview methods than from research using a validated rating scale or measurement instrument.

- Researchers need to describe the details of the data-gathering methods and the limitations of the data. These details, and scrupulous honesty and self-criticism on the part of the researcher, are necessary for others to decide how to use the research and also for the researcher to develop their research skills.

# Practical issues in planning and carrying out comparative health research

*If you fail to plan, you plan to fail.*

*The sources of quality research are skill, expertise and effort. The most important qualities of a researcher are humility, honesty and self-criticism. Practical resourcefulness, tolerance and persuasive diplomacy are just as important as technical skills for completing a successful comparative project.*

*You plan, and then life happens.*

## Introduction

The theme of this chapter is the need to plan and to be aware of the many practical problems and pitfalls of comparative research, and the purpose is to help researchers to plan and carry out a comparative research study. It will also be of use to those assessing research proposals or overseeing and managing research. It is primarily for a single researcher or a small team who are seeking to answer a question or test a hypothesis by making a comparison between items in one country or across countries, either by using available data or by collecting their own data. We also note practical issues in cross-area or cross-national collaborative studies involving researchers in different places.

The chapter describes a series of stages in a general research process, from initiation through to publication and dissemination of the results. This framework and the discussion aim to help researchers, sponsors and research supervisors to look ahead to some of the tasks that need to be done, and also to review progress and to replan at different stages.

It draws on the discussion of conceptual issues and methods given in earlier chapters and highlights the practical issues arising in each stage. It thus also serves as a summary of many of the subjects considered in the book. The following list details the items that need to be considered in planning a comparative study and in deciding the design and methods to use:

- *who* is the research for? (main users)

- what are the purposes, questions or hypotheses to be tested?

- what is the *'whole object'* to be compared and how will the specific objects be selected?

- *how many* items need to be compared to answer the research question?

- which *characteristics* of the different whole objects are to be compared, how are these characteristics defined and how many concepts/variables are to be studied?

- is the study to be *descriptive* only, or *explanatory* as well?

- will the study consider the *context*, and if so, which aspects to consider and why? (the theory about context-item influence)

- *data required*: which data are needed, and when and how often are these data to be collected? Are there data that have already been collected which can be used?

- *data gathering* and analysis methods

- *timing:* when are the results needed (e.g. to have the maximum influence on decision-making)? Are interim results needed or possible?

- *resources*: how much money, time and skills are available for the research, both those of the researchers and any collaborators? Are the resources fixed or negotiable?

## An overview of the phases of a comparative study

Many comparative studies run through the following phases, although not necessarily in this precise chronological sequence, especially the 'reviewing knowledge' phase. Note that this chronological sequence of research activities is not the same as the sequence and logic of presentation in a report. Each stage is discussed in more detail later in this chapter.

1 *Initiation*: taking action to seriously explore the feasibility, costs and possible benefits of making a comparison, and starting work to define an answerable question or hypothesis that could be tested. The initiator may be a researcher, a research user or a financial sponsor.

2 *Reviewing knowledge*: discovering and reviewing what is already known about the subject, identifying gaps and conflicting findings, and clarifying areas of certainty or theoretical controversy.

3 *Formulation*: deciding who the research is for, the aim and purpose, the specific question or hypothesis, the general and specific comparison to be made, the decisions it is to inform or the contribution it is to make (Chapter 4).

4 *Finalising research design details*: finalising design and the details of which specific comparisons are to be made, the data-gathering methods to use, how to use them and how to analyse the data (Chapter 5).

5 *Data collection and analysis*: gathering, recording and analysing data, using qualitative or quantitative methods or both (Chapter 6).

6 *Drawing conclusions and reporting*: building on the data analysis to make the conclusions and reporting what was discovered.

7 *Researcher self-review*: the researcher or team review the lessons for them from the research, and consider any methodological innovations or improvements they developed during the study.

A final introductory and practical point: planning is about deciding how best to use resources. A mistake that all researchers have made is to underestimate the time and skills needed for the study. When beginning a study it helps to have some idea of the time available, to look ahead at the phases listed above and then to draw a 'pie chart' with 'pie slices' for each of the seven phases, which gives an estimate of how much time to allocate to each phase (*see* Figure 7.1). This forces the researcher to recognise the time constraints and to prioritise by allocating percentages of the total time to each phase.

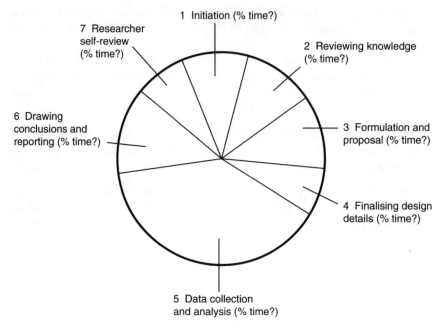

**Figure 7.1** Apportioning time or resources for each phase of the research

# Responsibilities and roles in the research process

Before considering issues in each of the seven phases, we first look at the roles and responsibilities of different parties in a research study:

- *researcher or research team*: the person or people carrying out the research – the latter may be sited in different areas or countries
- *users*: the people who will use the research, such as other researchers, practitioners, managers, policy-makers and citizens/patients
- *financial sponsor*: those paying for the research (which can be one or more users)
- *supervisor*: the manager or group overseeing the research (which can be a committee of users, sponsors, or a research or grants manager and expert advisors).

One of the most common reasons for practical problems to arise in a comparative study is the failure to agree the responsibilities of different parties, and this also delays action to respond to a problem during the research. Researchers, sponsors and others make assumptions about the roles and responsibilities of different parties, which may not be justified, especially if they are unfamiliar with the type of study that is being undertaken. Understanding and agreeing responsibilities in the early stages can prevent many common problems. Some of the different tasks, responsibilities and roles include:

- *The financial sponsor or their agent*: responsible for letting the researchers know when a decision will be made about whether to proceed, for providing finance of agreed amounts at agreed times in agreed ways and for giving agreed periods of notice of any termination of financing. Sometimes responsible for publishing or making the findings available.

- *The steering group or supervisor overseeing the research*: a group or individual responsible for giving advice and guidance to the researcher(s) during the study, and possibly for receiving and commenting on findings. Any rights to direct or overrule the researcher on any issues need to be agreed in this group's terms of reference.

- *The researcher(s) (project leader and staff)*: the main tasks and limits to their responsibilities need to be defined, especially if researchers at different sites are involved in a collaborative study, together with a timetable for the research and dates for reports and 'milestones', and budgetary and financial responsibilities.

- *Associated helpers (often health personnel)*: in some studies there is an agreement that health personnel or others will either co-operate or take an active role, possibly as full members of the research team. The expectations of them and the time for which they are assigned need to be agreed with them and their employers and need to be defined.

## Responsibilities in each phase of the research process

To further clarify responsibilities it helps to consider how decisions are to be made by different parties and who carries out different tasks in each phase of the research process. Table 7.1 gives a general illustration of how to use the model in this way to agree who makes which decisions and who is responsible for the different tasks.

**Table 7.1**: Clarification of responsibilities of different parties in each phase of a research study

| Phase | Sponsor/users/or collaborators Decides or does the task | Consults or does the task jointly | Lead researcher Decides or does the task |
|---|---|---|---|
| | Division of responsibilities | | |
| 1 Initiation | | | |
| 2 Reviewing knowledge | | Agree and state here: | |
| 3 Formulation | | • which tasks need to be done | |
| 4 Finalising research design details | | • who is responsible for what | |
| 5 Data collection and analysis | | • who has the right to be consulted or to make decisions | |
| 6 Drawing conclusions and reporting | | • how decisions are to be made | |
| 7 Researcher self-review | | | |

# Practical issues in each phase of a comparative study

This section looks at the practical issues to consider in each phase of a comparative study. The reader is also referred to the checklist for assessing and designing a comparative study in Appendix 2, which also raises issues that need to be considered in planning or assessing a proposal for a study.

## 1 Initiation

The initiation phase describes how the research originator takes his or her initial ideas and begins to explore the feasibility of conducting a study and the value of doing so. The originator may be a full-time researcher or a practitioner wishing to do research, and the motive may be curiosity or a known problem or gap in knowledge.

The originator may also be a manager, policy-maker or other practical user of the research. He or she may have an idea that comparative research on a subject would help them or others with a practical issue or problem, or would broaden their thinking about a subject they are working on. Their initial actions are often to 'sound out' other researchers informally, to find out whether research on the subject has been done, whether an invitation might be responded to, which researchers are most knowledgeable about the subject and who might be able to carry out or lead a project on the subject.

Questions to consider are:

- What are you interested in and why?

- What is the motive for doing the research?

- Who might benefit from it?

- What difference would it make to anyone to have the knowledge that might be created by the comparison?

- Why is a comparison required – could the knowledge be generated by a less expensive and less difficult approach?

The action part of initiation often involves seeking out potential sources of finance or other researchers and informally assessing whether a more detailed proposal is worth developing. There are sources of finance specifically for comparative research, or which are sympathetic to proposals for this type of research – these may be an international body or agencies within the originator's country. Finance is one resource, but there are others to consider, not least of which is the time of the originator or researcher. Will your employers support your spending time on such a study – how would it benefit your employing organisation and fit with its aims, if at all?

In some cases this informal initiation phase will lead directly to a proposal for formal approval or financing. More often, once the feasibility of a study is decided, this initiation phase is followed by a phase of reviewing existing knowledge and doing a literature search before making a formal proposal.

# 2 Reviewing knowledge

This phase refers to consulting experts and searching the databases and literature for what is already known about the subject and about previous comparisons, and reviewing the research. Sometimes the review is not the full extensive review which is needed for the final report, but is designed to be a broad overview to find out if research has already been done, or how to build on any previous research and define the question more precisely. One of the main purposes is to build up a background for defining answerable research questions or testable hypotheses and for showing the value of the research in the next phase of formulation and proposal. The aims are to identify gaps in knowledge, conflicting findings or theoretical controversy, and to clarify areas of uncertainty.

Descriptions of how to search computer and other databases for relevant published research are given in research methods texts, such as Edwards and Talbot (1994) and Gray (1997). Researchers can also carry out a meta-analysis or review of the research; details of how to do this are discussed in Gray (1997), NHSCR&D (1996) and, briefly, in St Leger *et al.* (1992, pp. 178–9).

*In all great quests there is a trial: the first in comparative research is defining the research question.*

# 3 Formulation and proposal

This phase of formulation refers to the work of drawing up an outline research proposal and plan. There is no sharp dividing line between initiation and formulation, but this third phase usually follows a decision to proceed to a formal proposal after having considered the general feasibility, cost and benefits of a study.

Formulation involves deciding and specifying who the research is for, its aim and purpose, the specific question or hypothesis, the general and specific comparison to be made, and the decisions it is to inform or the contribution it is to make. Formulating the research question and defining testable hypotheses is perhaps the most important and difficult part of the whole process (*see* Chapter 4, and also Black, 1993).

In most large-scale comparative studies, the sponsor will select a research team and a design from a number of proposals submitted to them. Sponsors are often not clear what they want and use the many proposals submitted to help them clarify exactly what it is they want studied and the questions to which they want answers. Usually the sponsor and the selected researchers will then negotiate further details in a planning phase. They will explore and negotiate the final purposes, design and details of the study before a formal contract is agreed. Researchers often have to help sponsors who know little about comparative research to define their questions and to educate them about what a research study can and cannot achieve.

Sometimes the researcher needs to carry out a feasibility assessment to find out more about the subject and to give the sponsor proposals for different types of study, including not doing one. Giving the sponsor a set of choices like this helps them to clarify what they want from the research and to understand more about the costs of different types of study.

The end result of the formulation phase should be a research plan which describes:

- who the study is for

- the purpose of the study and the one or more questions it aims to answer

- what is to be compared and the specific comparisons to be made

- the research design, including how many comparisons are to be made or how large the sample will be, and how the sample will be selected (e.g. for credibility, for statistical validity?)

- the methods used to gather and analyse data

- a time plan of activities and milestones

- the resources to be used and budget.

An important point in all research is a formal or informal contract between the researcher and sponsor (who may be the researcher's employer) about what the researcher will do. Contract agreement can follow a lengthy discussion about options and details, or it may be an agreement to carry out initial explorations in order to decide whether to make a comparison or to help formulate a detailed design.

# 4 Finalising details of design and methods

This phase follows a formal decision to proceed with the research. It involves the researcher planning the practical details and making detailed agreements with those with whom they will collaborate. These may be other researchers, or they may be people who will be supplying information or taking part in other aspects of the research.

Often the final decision to proceed is made some time after the initial formulation of the proposal and changes need to be made, or the proposal may be in general terms only and specific details need to be decided and agreed. The urge is always to rush into data collection, but even a small amount of time and thought at the final planning stage saves more time when collecting data and analysing it.

For some complex studies, a project management model is essential to planning and co-ordinating the different researchers and stages of the work. Project management is a technique developed in the construction sector, but which is now widely applied in health services (e.g. 'PRINCE') and scientific research programmes. Many management texts describe the techniques, and simple software such as 'Microsoft Project' can help even the solo researcher to plan details, highlight critical decision points and times, and manage their study over time.

# 5 Data collection and analysis

In the phase of data collection and analysis the researcher uses quantitative or qualitative methods to collect and analyse data. They may use existing data sources, such as government statistics, patient medical records or service documents. Or they may create and use their own data-gathering instruments. Even if they are using secondary data, researchers need to carefully plan the timing and practical details of data collection, and how they will minimise the weaknesses and maximise the strengths of their chosen methods. These issues were discussed in Chapter 6 when considering observation, interviewing, questionnaires, surveys, measurement and using existing data. Appendix 3 gives a checklist for assessing data quality, which also helps when planning data collection. The issues to consider in planning which data to collect, and how and when to collect the data, are listed below:

- should there be a small pilot test of the data-gathering methods (e.g. if making a survey)?

- are pilot tests required in the different populations or sites to be compared?

- how to get access to the people to be interviewed or to service documents and records

- how often and when do the data need to be collected?

- how will data be recorded in order to make analysis easier?

- is there a need for expert advice or for a specialist to undertake some of the data collection?

- what does previous research that used this method teach us about how to maximise validity and reliability, and have the methods we plan to use been validated in one, or all, of the study populations or sites?

- how do we get co-operation from service personnel and patients, if they are to be involved?

- what is the best way to introduce ourselves as researchers to different parties? Do we have to be careful about what we say so as to minimise biasing what people might tell us?

- have we considered the ethical issues of data collection and reporting, such as protecting privacy, seeking permission, respecting cultural and other sensitivities?

A task that is often neglected when planning research is to look ahead to how data will be analysed and then drawn together in a report in a way that will answer the research question(s). The dividing line between data collection and data analysis is arbitrary, because data collection often involves a recording method which is itself a form of analysis, such as a pre-structured set of questions for an interview. So, too, is the line between analysis and drawing conclusions: when considering alternative explanations the researchers may go back to the data to reanalyse it to test other possible associations (referred to as 'snooping', 'fishing' and 'hunting' by Slevin and Stuart, 1978). Such a practice is frowned on in experimental research which requires that the hypotheses are stated before the data gathering, rather than after.

# 6 Drawing conclusions and reporting

This phase involves looking back critically over the data gathering and analysis and stating all the limitations of the methods and data. Drawing conclusions involves considering all possible alternative explanations for the findings and stating the degree of certainty of the findings. When planning, anticipate alternative explanations and, if possible, design the research to exclude them.

There will be pressures on the researchers to state practical conclusions and recommendations, and where these are stated, the report needs to point out what 'leaps', if any, are made from the findings to the practical conclusions. It helps when planning and when part way through a study to look ahead at the questions that different parties will have of the study, and to think about whether the study can answer these and with what degree of certainty. In planning a study, researchers need to think about how they can best communicate their findings. By considering early on how to present their report, researchers may then look at the data analysis methods and may decide to use different methods which give more direct answers to the original research questions and to those which their audiences may raise. The research plan should also record agreements with the sponsor about publication rights and whether sponsors or others would be able to veto publication of any details, as well as who should deal with any requests for copies of the research report.

*Incomprehensibility is not a necessary requirement of scrupulous research. The difference between a successful and unsuccessful comparative study is often the ability of the researcher to communicate their findings and the limitations to non-experts.*

Increasingly, the role of researchers is to help users to incorporate the research information into their decisions and actions. However, researchers need to be able to judge when they are being drawn into decisions that others should be making, and to point out when the evidence is being used to support actions which the evidence does not justify. In deciding action, users of research have many issues to consider and other facts, apart from the findings of the research.

Researchers need to make clear the limitations of the evidence and what the evidence does and does not conclusively show and how the researchers think that this relates to the decisions to be made. They need to clearly explain problems which arose during the study which affected the evidence, such as poor response rate to questionnaires, problems in making valid comparisons (see Chapter 4), and any other relevant unanticipated and uncontrollable changes during the study which may affect the findings. Some of these issues and predictable problems should have been thought through when the study was designed.

---

**Box 7.1: Four questions for managers or policy-makers deciding the practical actions that might follow from a comparison**

1 Is there a difference? (Is it a valid difference?)

2 What is the cause (or explanation)?

3 Can we do anything about it?

4 Is it a political priority to do something about it?

# 7 Researcher self-review

The final phase is where the researcher or team spend time reviewing what they have learnt from the study. One aim is to draw lessons on how to conduct future comparative research and for self-development as a health researcher. The best learning is through reflecting on experience and relating this to texts on methods. Researchers should compare what happened during the study to their original plan and proposal, and consider the strengths and weaknesses of their methods and what they might be able to use in future research. Other aims for a review are to consider the contribution the study could make to comparative health theory and methodology, and whether findings could be generalised and would be of interest to other researchers and health service personnel. There are many reasons why researchers rarely allocate time to carry out a review. If researchers are likely to carry out comparative research again or are in a group that specialises in this work, then there are particularly strong reasons for building into the plan and timetable both the time and finance for a review.

The above discussion of the seven phases should not be taken as an implication that planning and conducting a comparative study are questions of following a checklist sequence. Certainly some research is more like immersing oneself in a sea of questions to find where the current is taking one. However, looking ahead is essential for all types of research, and there are many predictable problems that need to be considered and prevented or planned for.

*Tolerance, patience and persuasive diplomacy are more important qualities for leading a cross-national research project than technical research skills.*

## Conclusions

- Many comparative research studies follow a similar sequence of seven phases in the planning and conduct of the study: initiation; reviewing knowledge; formulation and proposal; finalising design; data collection and analysis; drawing conclusions and reporting; and researcher self-review.

- This framework helps both researchers and research supervisors to look ahead, alerts them to possible problems and gives a background for assessing proposals, negotiating a contract and for managing the research. It also reminds researchers of the need to plan realistically how their time is to be used.

- Technical knowledge is not enough to plan a comparative research study or to deal with practical problems when they do occur. Some problems are common and predictable, but others cannot be foreseen. Experienced researchers try to reduce the chances of the unpredictable damaging the study, and they have a repertoire of tactics to deal with the more common problems that are likely to arise.

- How the researcher foresees and responds to practical problems that arise when carrying out the study can significantly affect the validity and utilisation of the findings.

- The single most common cause of many problems is failure to agree the responsibilities of different parties. These responsibilities need to be agreed for each of the phases of the research process, especially if it involves researchers at different sites or in different countries.

- Researchers will find checklists for assessing research useful when they are planning a study (e.g. Appendix 2), because these highlight potential weaknesses of a study that can be corrected in the planning stage.

- Researchers have different views about whether they have any responsibility for encouraging the utilisation of their findings. All have a duty to state the limitations of the findings and to resist pressures to recommend actions that cannot be justified by the findings or which require others to take other factors into consideration.

- Researchers need to be aware of the politics of research, of unacknowledged agendas, likely problems in access to data sources and co-operation, about how to build credibility and trust, and of how best to communicate their findings.

- At the end of the process, researchers need to build in time and finance for self-review and for publishing innovations in methodology to develop themselves and the transdiscipline of comparative health research.

- The only things that are certain in cross-national research are that some collaborators will be late with the data (or not provide it at all) and that there will be misunderstandings. The skill is to minimise these problems, and to learn from one's mistakes.

# Appendix I
# Definitions

*Action research*: a systematic investigation which aims to contribute to scientific knowledge as well as solve a practical problem.

*Audit*: an investigation into whether an activity meets explicit standards or procedures as defined by an auditing document. The auditing process can be carried out by external auditors or internally for self-review, and can use external ready-made audit standards or internally developed standards. Medical and clinical audit is using pre-existing standards or setting standards, comparing practice with standards and changing practice if necessary, and is usually carried out internally for self-review and improvement. Peer audit can use already-existing standards or practitioners can develop their own, but usually practitioners adapt existing standards to their own situation.

*'Blinding' – single-blinded trial*: the people in the control and experimental groups (subjects) do not know which group they are in.

*'Blinding' – double-blinded trial*: neither the subjects nor the service-providers know which group is the experimental group and which is the control.

*Boundary*: (a) that which separates the 'whole object' from its context and allows differentiation of the whole object from the context and definition of it; (b) a term used to describe how the context is mediated to the item (e.g. causes operate on the whole object through a boundary).

*Case–control study*: a restrospective observational study of people or organisations with a particular characteristic ('cases') compared to those which do not have this characteristic ('controls'), to find out possible causes or influences which could explain the characteristic.

*Case study*: 'attempts to examine a contemporary phenomenon in its real-life context, especially when the boundaries between context and phenomenon are not clearly evident' (Yin, 1981).

*Characteristic*: a concept, dimension or variable which describes an aspect of the entity that is compared – death, disease, levels of management, financing method, etc.

*Cohort*: a group of people, usually sharing one or more characteristics, who are followed over time to find out what happens to them.

*Community diagnosis*: a process of collecting, describing, analysing and disseminating information about health and its determinants in a community.

*Confounding factors or variables*: something other than the intervention which could influence the measured outcome. Alternative definition: 'confounding arises when an observed association between two variables is due to the action of a third factor' (Crombie, 1996).

*Context*: the 'environment' surrounding the whole object, which is usually different in different areas. The context is conceptualised by the researchers in terms of different factors or characteristics of context.

*Continuous quality improvement*: an approach for ensuring that staff continually improve work processes by using proven quality methods to discover and resolve the causes of quality problems in a systematic way.

*Control group or control site*: a group of people or an organisation that do not get the intervention. The research compares them to the experimental group or site, which gets the intervention. People are randomly allocated to either group, or, if this is not possible, the control group or site is 'matched' with the experimental group.

*Cost-benefit*: valuing the consequences of a programme in money terms, so as to compare the assessed value with the actual costs. A range of benefits are valued in money terms.

*Cost description*: measurement of the costs of one thing, or of more than one, in a way which allows a comparison of costs. (A 'partial' economic evaluation looks at only one intervention and does not make an explicit comparison.)

*Cost-effectiveness*: the effectiveness or consequences as shown on one measure, for the cost (e.g. lives saved, cases of diseases avoided, years of healthy life). No attempt is made to value the consequences – it is assumed that the output is of value. Used to compare the different costs of using different ways to achieve the same end result.

*Cost minimisation*: assumes that the differences in outcome produced by the alternatives are not significant, and calculates the cost of each alternative with the purpose of discovering which is the lowest cost.

*Cost-utility:* considers the utility of the end result to the patient for the cost. Often uses the quality-adjusted life year (QALY) measure (Drummond *et al.*, 1987). Measures consequences in time units adjusted by health utility weights (i.e. states of health associated with outcome are valued relative to each other). More complex than cost-effectiveness.

*Criterion*: a comparison against which we judge the evaluated – effectiveness is often such a criterion.

*Culture:* the combination of laws, customs, rules, language and ideas shared by a group of people and through which individuals express, understand and give meaning to their own and others' experiences.

*Data-gathering method*: a method used to gather data about an item, and to gather data about the context to the item.

*Descriptive CHR*: research to discover the presence or absence of an item in different places or to describe similarities and differences (e.g. statistical comparisons, some survey comparisons, some case studies).

*Design*: the overall research design, including sampling and how the items are compared.

*Ecological correlation*: a correlation between factors or variables which were discovered when studying a population. Such correlations might not necessarily apply to individuals – assuming that they do is an 'ecological fallacy'.

*Empirical*: the collection of data about the subject studied, in order to test hypotheses or to build up conceptualisations about it.

*Empiricism*: an approach to research which holds that the real world exists independently of the observer's concepts about it and can be apprehended directly: 'the facts speak for themselves'.

*Evaluation:* a comparative assessment of the value of an intervention, in relation to criteria and using systematically collected and analysed data, in order to decide how to act.

*Evidence-based medicine*: 'the conscientious, explicit, and judicious use of current best evidence in making decisions about the care of individual patients. The practice of EBM means integrating individual clinical expertise with best available external clinical evidence from systematic research' (Sackett *et al.*, 1996).

*Experimental CHR*: aims to test hypotheses by intervening in one or more places and by using statistical methods.

*Explanatory CHR:* research which aims to understand, interpret or explain why similarities or differences occur (e.g. many epidemiological studies, some case studies).

*'Genotypical' CHR*: research interested in discovering deep-level similarities in the phenomena in different areas or countries, despite superficial differences ('the items look different, but there are underlying similarities').

*Item:* a general term for that which is compared. The item may be a characteristic, or it may be a process. The item compared may also be an entity, as, for example, in an exploratory study to discover any similarities and differences in an entity found in two or more places.

*Management technology transfer*: transferring management technologies from one setting to another by identifying management methods which could be used to solve problems or improve management actions in another place, and by using methods for adapting and applying these methods sensitively to a particular local setting.

*Matching*: ensuring that people (or organisations) in the experimental and control groups (or sites) are the same, in all the characteristics which could affect the outcome of the intervention which is given to the experimental group or site.

*Monitoring*: continuous supervision of an activity to check whether plans and procedures are being followed. (Audit is a sub-type of the wider activity of monitoring.)

*Operationalisation*: converting something general (e.g. a criterion) into something specific which can be measured or about which data can be collected (e.g. operationalising the concept of pain in one or more rating scales of pain).

*Organisational audit*: an external inspection of aspects of a service, in comparison to established standards, and a review of an organisation's arrangements to control and assure the quality of its products or services. Audits use criteria (or 'standards') against which auditors judge elements of a service's planning, organisation, systems and performance.

*Outcome measure*: a measure of an important predicted effect of an intervention on the target person or population. Outcome: the difference an intervention makes to the person, population or organisation which is the target of the intervention.

*Phenomenological CHR*: seeks to understand and interpret the meanings which people give to events and experiences in different places.

*'Phenotypical' CHR*: research which examines superficially similar items to discover deep-level differences ('the items looks the same, but there are underlying differences').

*Placebo:* something which the subjects of an intervention think is an intervention, but which has no known 'active ingredient' (used to control for effects which may be caused only by subjects thinking that they are receiving an intervention).

*Positivism*: an approach to research which holds that increasingly certain knowledge can be created by testing hypotheses, which are derived from theory, by using experimental methods. Does not hold, like empiricism does, that reality can be apprehended directly without concepts, but does seek to refute hypotheses empirically by gathering data using pre-observational categories.

*Power* (of experimental research design): the probability of correctly rejecting the null hypothesis of no difference in outcome between intervention and control groups, where an intervention effect exists (Armatage & Berry, 1987).

*Prevention*: actions to prevent the occurrence of a disease, or to arrest its progress and reduce its effects once it is established. Primary prevention aims to prevent the initial occurrence of a disease. Secondary prevention aims to stop or slow existing disease through early detection. Tertiary prevention aims to reduce relapses and to prevent chronicity and hospitalisation.

*Process comparison*: a comparison of changes over time in two or more entities, or a comparison of a sequence of activities carried out by or to an entity.

*Prospective study or evaluation*: designing a study or an evaluation and then collecting data while the intervention is happening, and usually also before and after the intervention.

*Quality*: meeting the health needs of those most in need at the lowest cost and within regulations (Øvretveit, 1992). The quality of a service is measured in terms of the three dimensions of patient, professional and management quality. Does the service give patients what they want, what professionals think they need, without wasting resources and within regulations?

*Quality accreditation*: a certification through an external evaluation of whether a practitioner, equipment or a service meets standards which are thought to contribute to quality processes and outcomes.

*Quality assurance*: a general term for activities and systems for monitoring and improving quality. Quality assurance involves, but is more than, measuring quality and evaluating quality.

*Randomisation*: allocating people in a random way to an experimental or a control group. The purpose is to try to ensure that the people (or organisations) with characteristics which might affect the outcome are allocated evenly to both groups. If any differences between the two groups are more than chance differences, then these differences are likely to be significant if enough people were included and they were randomly allocated. Randomisation is superior to matching because there are many known and unknown characteristics which may influence outcome.

*Randomised controlled trial*: an experiment where one group gets the intervention and another group does not, and people are assigned to both groups in a random way. (*Control group*: a group of people who do not get the intervention or are not subjected to a hypothesised causal influence.)

*Research – basic or pure*: the use of scientific methods which are appropriate for discovering valid knowledge of a phenomenon for the purpose of contributing to scientific knowledge about the subject.

*Retrospective study or evaluation*: looking into the past for evidence about the subject or intervention. ('Concurrent' means at the same time.)

*Review*: a single or regular assessment of an activity, which may or may not compare the activity to an explicit plan, criteria or standards. (Most audits or monitoring are types of review.)

*Self-evaluation*: practitioners or teams who evaluate their own practice so as to improve it.

*Sensitivity*: the ability of a test to detect all true positives, or of a measure to detect changes in the phenomena being measured.

*Specificity*: the ability of a test to identify true negatives.

*Sponsor*: those who initiate or pay for the research.

*Standardised mortality ratio (SMR)*: the ratio of the number of deaths observed in the study population to the number of deaths expected if it had the same rate structure as the standard population.

*Subjectivism*: an approach to research which holds that an explanation of both an individual and a group act must make reference to the subjective meaning given to the act by the actors. Views human beings as meaning-creating creatures, with choice, and holds that social phenomena can only be understood in context and by reference to culture.

*User*: one who makes use of or acts on a comparative research study.

*Validity – internal validity*: the validity of the conclusions of research for the particular people or entities studied, or the validity of an evaluation experiment, for example in being able to show whether or not the intervention has an effect or the size of the effect.

*Validity – external validity*: the ability of a research study or evaluation experiment to show that the findings would also apply elsewhere or when the intervention is applied in another setting.

*Variable – confounding variable(s)*: any variable which influences the dependent variable or outcome but was not considered or controlled for in the study. Alternative definition: 'confounding arises when an observed association between two variables is due to the action of a third factor' (Crombie, 1996).

*Variable – dependent variable(s)*: the outcome variable or end result of a treatment, service or policy which is the subject of the study (e.g. cancer mortality, patient satisfaction, resources consumed by a service), and which might be associated with or even caused by other (independent) variables. The study tests for associations between the dependent (outcome) variable and the independent variables.

*Variable – extraneous variable(s)*: variables not considered in the theory or model used in the study.

*Variable – independent variable(s)*: a variable whose possible effect on the dependent variable is examined. (Something which may cause the outcome and which is tested in the research.)

*Variable – mediating variable(s)*: other variables which could affect the dependent variable or outcome, which the research tries to control for in design or in statistical analysis (e.g. outcome).

*Whole 'object' or 'entity' which is compared*: two or more individuals, populations, organisations, systems, policies or interventions to organisation.

# Appendix 2
# Check sheet for assessing a comparative research study

*This check sheet can also be used to assess a proposal for a study or to help to improve the design and planning of a study.*

## 1 Question definition

(a) Did the study sufficiently consider previous research and draw on this to define the question or the hypothesis? (Are any important studies in the field not considered?)

(b) Does the study define a clear and specific question which is answerable, or a testable hypothesis? (Are there too many questions or hypotheses to be addressed properly in a single study?)

(c) Is the question or hypothesis to be tested significant, of interest and likely to help people make better informed decisions?

(d) Does the study give a justification for the cost and efforts of a comparative study rather than another type of study?

## 2 Concept comparability

(a) Does the research define the whole object and the characteristic(s) of it which are to be compared in different areas?

(b) Does the research consider the possible reasons for items in different areas not being comparable?

(c) If the research involves data gathering from subjects, does the study adequately justify using the same concept in different populations if the concept does not have the same meaning to subjects in these different populations?

## 3 Design quality

(a) Is the design clearly described, together with the timescale with dates showing the main research activities and when, and over which time period, the data were gathered?

(b) Data sample/selection: does the study describe the sample of people or 'units' from which data are collected (data sources) and justify selecting these sources in relation to the research question?

(c) Are there too few or too many items compared in order to answer the research question or test the hypothesis?

(d) In practice: is the design practical and capable of being carried out by reasonably well-trained researchers with the amount of resources which could be expected for this type of study?

(e) In theory: is the sample and the design able to answer the research question or test the hypothesis, if the study is carried out perfectly?

## 4 Data-gathering methods and data quality

(a) For a study of this type in *one* place, are the methods suitable for gathering data about a subject of this type?

(b) Does the research use valid operational definitions of the concept(s)?

(c) Are the operational definitions the same for *all* the data gathering, in different areas or populations?

(d) Are all possible differences considered in how the data were collected in different places or for different populations?

(e) Does the study describe the precautions for ensuring that the data were collected in the same way in different places or populations, and are these precautions adequate for ensuring the reliability of the data?

(f) Are the data-gathering methods appropriate for answering the question or the hypothesis to be tested?

(g) Could there be bias in the data which the study (a) does not recognise, or (b) is not able to correct for?

(h) Are there any limitations of the data-gathering methods or of the data which the study does not describe or does not take into account?

# 5 Data analysis

(a) Does the study use analysis techniques which are normally accepted as the best to use for this type of data and question, or justify the analysis techniques which are used?

(b) From the description in the study of how the analysis methods were applied, is there any evidence that these methods were applied either correctly or incorrectly?

(c) Is there a clear and acceptable description of any adjustments made for possible differences in how the data were collected in different places or for different populations?

# 6 Conclusions/recommendations

If all the above are adequate, then:

(a) Does the research show the logical links between questions, design, methods, data, analysis and conclusions?

(b) If explanations or interpretations are given, are there any possible alternative explanations or interpretations which are not considered?

(c) Is sufficient justification given for rejecting alternative explanations or interpretations?

(d) Are there conclusions which are not supported by the evidence, and, if so, is this stated?

(e) Generally, are there any reasons to doubt the conclusions drawn from the analysis, or the justifications given for recommendations?

# Appendix 3
# Check sheet for assessing the data used in a comparative research study

## 1 How reliable are the data?

- What precautions were used in the research to ensure and maximise the reliability of data in *one* population or *one* area? (e.g. interviewer training)

- Could there be consistency errors in data collected for *one* population or in *one* area (systematic bias or random) which are introduced by the data-gathering method?

- Were the same methods used in the different areas or for the different populations?

- Would others using the same methods have collected the same data?

- What are the particular ways of assessing the reliability of data gathered using this method and how far do the data meet these criteria?

## 2 How valid are the data?

- Are the concepts which define the type of data required discussed, as well as their applicability in different areas or populations?

- Are the theoretical links between the concepts and the measure (or data) described? (Discussion of 'operationalisation' of concepts)

- If the study used a standard data-gathering method, did it use the techniques for ensuring validity which are usually used for this method?

# 3 Sampling

- Are the areas, populations or institutions selected for the study described?

- Was the sampling method justified?

- What assumptions are made if generalisations are made from this sample?

# 4 Method of analysis

- Is the method of analysis described?

- What are the usual methods of analysis used for this type of data for this type of study?

- How well were these analysis methods applied?

# 5 Presentation of evidence

- Are raw data presented or available for inspection?

# 6 Credibility

- If the evidence points to necessary changes, will the evidence be credible to the people who have to change?

# 7 Ethics

- Were the data collected and reported in an ethical way? (e.g. patients anonymous, were documents public or 'cleared'?)

# Appendix 4
# Examples of comparative health research studies

| Type of study<br>Comparison of | Sub-type<br>Comparison of | Details | Reference |
|---|---|---|---|
| **1 POPULATION HEALTH NEEDS** | | | |
| **Needs of populations in developing countries** | | Study describes methods for rapid assessment in tropical disease research – the methods can give information on health status, health impact, health services and health behaviour | Vlassoff & Tanner (1992) |
| **Needs of populations in urban areas of Western countries** | | Study describes and illustrates, with an example, the use of rapid assessment for assessing needs in UK urban areas | Ong (1993) |
| **Mental health needs and demands** | Areas in five Nordic countries | Study of hidden psychiatric morbidity and prevalence of psychiatric illness in 1281 patients consulting GPs in a Nordic multicentre study | Fink *et al.* (1995); Munk-Jørgensen *et al.* (1997) |
| **Primary health care needs** | Patients of five GP practices | A survey of patients registered with five Scottish general medical practices ($n$ = 3478) to gather data about patients' reported health problems and other data. | Hopton & Dlugolecka (1995) |
| **Health needs-related socio-economic indicators** | Index of socio-economic status for health comparisons | Considers existing data in Canada on socio-economic attributes of geographical areas, and mortality and morbidity data. The study presents a method for selecting and combining measures of area socio-economic characteristics to produce a composite index which is of use for comparative health research. It compares this index with deprivation indices in the UK which also show strong associations with measures of health status and service utilisation | Frohlich & Mustard (1996) |

**For other general statistical comparisons see section 9 (below)**

| Type of study Comparison of | Sub-type Comparison of | Details | Reference |
|---|---|---|---|
| 2  HEALTH STATES, BEHAVIOUR AND ATTITUDES | | | |
| **Death (mortality rates)** | Databases – raw statistics (classified by cause of death, some also by age and sex) | Comparison of mortality by major categories, as well as morbidity and many other health care service comparisons, with simple summary comments in English and Danish | NOMESCO (1996) |
| | | Similar to above, but includes non-health comparisons (e.g. mortality in 52 categories of cause, mortality from cardiovascular disease for six age categories, male and female) | NCM (1995) |
| | | Europe | Eurostat (1992); WHO (1992) |
| | | OECD countries | OECD (1993a,b) |
| | | Eastern Europe | Boys et al. (1991) |
| **Avoidable mortality** | Mostly raw statistics | Nordic | NOMESCO (1996); NCM (1995) |
| | | Comparable rates in Europe of avoidable mortality | WHO (1992) |
| | Cardiovascular mortality | Comparison and discussion of differences and possible causes | Rosen & Thelle (1996) |
| | Cancer mortality in central Europe | Comparison of changes in mortality from major cancer sites and all cancer sites combined, in six central Europe countries. WHO mortality database used and data analysed for 13–17 birth cohorts | Evstifeeva et al. (1997) |
| **Disease (morbidity rates)** | Nordic and European | Comparative disease rates may be found in the same databases as for mortality rates: see above for Nordic, European and OECD | NOMESCO (1996); NCM (1995); Eurostat (1992); WHO (1992); OECD (1993a) |
| | Explanations for differences in health in Europe | Uses WHO and European Union databases to compare health in 12 European countries, and considers their differences in terms of a model of determinants of health. Short discussion of data limitations and the need for European standardisation | Schaapveld et al. (1995) |
| | Coronary heart disease | CHD in 11 900 men of Japanese ancestry living in Japan, Hawaii and California, related to risk factors. The study showed that, 'the culture in which the individual is raised affects his likelihood of manifesting coronary heart disease in adult life', and that the relationship of culture of upbringing to CHD was independent of risk factors | Marmot & Syme (1976); see also Marmot et al. (1975) |

| Type of study Comparison of | Sub-type Comparison of | Details | Reference |
|---|---|---|---|
| **Health expectancy** | Databases – raw statistics | Life expectancy in the Nordic countries | NOMESCO (1996); NCM (1995) |
| | | International comparison of the number of years an average person can expect to live in good health during his or her lifetime | Boshuizen et al. (1994) |
| | Health expectancy indicator | Discussion of an HE measure for Europe and a survey of policy-makers' views about the use of such a measure. HE combines mortality with morbidity data | van de Water et al. (1996) |
| **Health perceptions** | Health and illness (subjective perception) comparisons between populations | Self-reported health. Special survey of 12 EU member states: Of different socio-economic groups Related to death rate | CEC (1988) |
| | | New 'perceived health' indicator for Europe only recently developed, but only regional values known | Schaapveld et al. (1995) |
| | Long-term illness | Comparison of self-reported health from interviews of 23 864 Swedish and foreign-born people in Sweden. Study controlled for social material and lifestyle factors and examined association between ethnicity and limiting long-term illness | Sundquist & Johansson (1997) |
| | Quality of life | The 'International Quality of Life' (IQOLA) project uses the SF-36 instrument to compare the outcomes of health care delivery systems and of specific treatments (presentation by John Ware at the fifth annual conference of the European Public Health association, 1996, London) | |
| **Health-related behaviour** | Cancer-related | Behaviour and attitudes in Europe | CEC (1988) |
| | Alcohol consumption | Europe | WHO (1992) |
| | Tobacco consumption | For adult populations in 1990 | World Bank (1993) |
| | Alcoholism | Forty authors from nine different countries discuss issues and report on research arising out of the Epidemiological Catchment Area study. This study used a standardised psychiatric diagnostic interview which gave good agreement amongst psychiatrists about the psychiatric disease. The book considers the cultural aspects of alcohol consumption and the prevalence, symptom frequency and onset and course of alcohol dependence in nine countries. (e.g. USA 7.9%, Taiwan 1.5 %) | Helzer & Canino (1992) |

| Type of study Comparison of | Sub-type Comparison of | Details | Reference |
|---|---|---|---|
| | Nutrition | For example, per capital annual consumption of vegetables, meat, dairy products, calories, etc. | Eurostat (1992); OECD (1993) |
| | Sleep | Comparison of subject-reported sleep problems and other variables in 453 Norwegians and 450 Russians living in the Norwegian and Russian areas of the Svalbard region | Nilssen *et al.* (1997) |
| | Suicide | Comparison within Sweden of the variation in suicide rates of data of immigration, ethnicity, age, sex and marital status, using central 'Cause of Death Register' and 1985 Swedish census | Johansson *et al.* (1997) |
| | Parasuicide | Comparison of medically treated parasuicide incidence in five Nordic countries and risk factors, as well as follow-up comparisons of personal and social characteristics predictive of future suicidal behaviour | Stiles *et al.* (1993) |
| **Health-related attitudes** | Children's attitudes | Comparison of the health perceptions, behaviour and attitudes of school-aged children in 19 European countries and Canada and Greenland, using questionnaires to about 1300 respondents in each country | WHO (1996) |
| 3 TREATMENTS | **(for screening and prevention see section 4 below)** | | |
| **Pharmaceuticals** | Prescription of systemic antibiotics | Differences in rate of prescription between the Nordic countries (Finland defined daily doses 3 times higher than Denmark and Norway) | NOMESCO (1996) |
| **Surgery** | Variations in surgical rates | Comparison of rates for common surgical procedures in New England, England and Norway, using data from hospital data reported to regional government or regional data centres, which was standardised for age and sex | McPherson *et al.* (1982) |
| | Variations in surgical rates | Using NOMESCO data, the study compares rates between three or more Nordic countries of appendectomy, cholesystectomy, disc, hip, hysterectomy, breast cancer, prostatectomy, and Caesarian section surgery | Madsen (1996) |

| Type of study<br>Comparison of | Sub-type<br>Comparison of | Details | Reference |
|---|---|---|---|
| **Various medical care practices** | International differences | Overview of international comparisons of medical care utilisation, and discussion of the usefulness of such comparisons in understanding clinical decision-making, their purposes, and methodological and policy issues involved | McPherson (1989) |

4  Services and health organisations

| Type of study<br>Comparison of | Sub-type<br>Comparison of | Details | Reference |
|---|---|---|---|
| **Use of health services** | Use of preventative health care services | For Europe, use of cervical smear test, % of women at least once in 1991 | CEC (1991) |
|  |  | Immunisation rate, % of children in first year with third dose of DPT (1990) | World Bank (1993) |
|  | Primary health care – use of by patients with psychiatric problems | Comparison of the use of psychiatric outpatient services in the USA and Ontario, using data from two general population surveys which used identical assessments of need for services, questions about their use, and other indicators | Kessler *et al.* (1997) |
| **Home care services** | Comparison of Danish and Swedish home care services | Action research comparison of services in Sweden and Denmark | Lewinter (1997) |
| **Activities** | Referrals from primary to secondary care | Comparison of referral rates in 15 European countries by collecting information about 30 consecutive referrals by a number of GPs in each country | RCGP (1992) |
| **Structure** | Hospital medical director roles | Describes different models of the role of medical middle managers in English hospitals. Original model derives from Johns Hopkins management structure. The concepts and framework have been used for other cross-national comparisons | IHSM (1990) |
| **Financing** |  | Reforms to hospital financing systems – international comparison | Wiley (1992) |
| **Performance** | Costs – private vs public USA | In-country (USA) comparison of costs of care and administration of for-profit and other hospitals, using HCFA-provided data tapes of hospital expenses, which were linked to HCFA's Medicare minimum dataset for 1992–93 | Woolhandler & Himmelstein (1997) |

| Type of study Comparison of | Sub-type Comparison of | Details | Reference |
|---|---|---|---|
| | Health personnel payment systems | Comparison of pay determination systems in UK and USA health services | Buchan (1997) |
| | Activity and outputs | A comparison of Scottish hospitals for 1991 using data describing in-patient or day-case discharges from gynaecological units as well as data from Scottish Morbidity Records Form 1. The study shows the importance when making comparisons between outcomes of taking into account characteristics of patients, diagnostic case mix and the social circumstances of the area | Leyland & Boddy (1997) |
| | Outcomes | Hospital mortality: methods used in comparisons and one study of 22 north-west London hospitals using in-hospital mortality rates adjusted by disease severity and calculated on the basis of both admissions and episodes | Mckee & Hunter (1995) |
| | Quality | Different US and UK systems for comparing patient satisfaction and outcomes, summarised in Øvretveit (1996a) | Øvretveit (1996a) |
| | | Description of the Maryland Hospital Quality Indicator comparisons project | Thompson et al. (1997) |
| | | Comparison of patient satisfaction and outcomes in Norwegian hospitals | Guldvog et al. (1995) |
| **History** | Home births and maternity services | Historical comparison of changes in home and hospital births in Sweden and Denmark, using historical documents and government statistics | Vallgårda (1996) |
| | Methodology – problems with the UK 'labour productivity index' | Example of a study which looks at the problems calculating and using a composite performance indicator in the UK – the labour productivity index. This index combines data on activity such as inpatients, outpatients, health visitor contacts, etc., which are weighted using the national average cost of producing one unit of the various types of activity, and then combined into an overall index by multiplying each by average cost, adding these and dividing by the total number of employees. Many issues are similar for other composite indicators | Appleby (1996) |

| Type of study<br>Comparison of | Sub-type<br>Comparison of | Details | Reference |
|---|---|---|---|
| **5 INTERVENTIONS TO HEALTH ORGANISATIONS** | | | |
| | Comparison of hospital quality programmes | Eight UK quality programmes compared, including two in non-health organisations | Joss & Kogan (1995) |
| | | Six hospital programmes compared in Norway (the Norwegian TQM pilot). The study described the quality programmes as they were developed and the experience of each hospital on a number of dimensions. The researchers gathered data from middle managers about their experience and perceptions, using a standard semi-structured interview, and collected any evidence which was collected by the hospitals about the effects of the programmes | Øvretveit (1996b)<br><br>Øvretveit & Aslaksen (1998) |
| | Comparison of quality assessment systems | Organisational audit, quality awards, quality systems | Øvretveit (1994b) |
| | Comparison of accreditation methods | USA, Australia and Canada before 1988 | Sketris (1988) |
| | | USA, Canada, Australia, UK | Scrivens (1995) |
| **6 HEALTH SYSTEMS** | | | |
| | Statistical comparisons – OECD | | OECD (1990; 1993b) |
| | Financing | Comparison of financing and delivery in OECD countries | OECD (1987) |
| | Nordic health systems | Most recent comprehensive description of each Nordic health system, by country experts, and comparison of aspects (e.g. patient co-payments), with overviews | Alban & Christiansen (1995) |
| | Financing – GP payments | A description of GP remuneration systems in Australia, Canada, Denmark, Norway and the UK found large differences, but similarities between countries in unclarity about the objectives of general practice | Kristiansen & Mooney (1993) |
| | Organisation and management | OECD, WHO, World Bank and Nordic Council descriptions | |

| Type of study<br>Comparison of | Sub-type<br>Comparison of | Details | Reference |
|---|---|---|---|
| | Equity | In financing and delivery of health care based on a 10 European country project. Proposes a common methodology for studying equity, and discovered three different profiles for how health care payments rise as a proportion of income as income rises ('progressivity profiles') | Doorslaer *et al.* (1994) |
| | Citizens' views | 'Eurobarometer' survey of citizens' views in 15 European countries of satisfaction with health system, views about reforms, and attitudes towards spending on health care | Mossialos (1997) |
| | | Details of methods in Reif & Ingelhart (1991) | Reif & Ingelhart (1991) |
| | Dimensions for comparison | Broad comparison of system performance in terms of overall cost control, efficiency of service delivery, equity in access, and responsiveness in Sweden, Holland, West Germany, USA and Canada | Ham *et al.* (1990) |
| | | Conceptual discussion of comparison of different types of equity and choice in health care systems and reforms | Øvretveit (1994a) |
| | Methodology – typologies of health systems | A 'modular' approach to analysing health systems, with concepts of modules of population needs, manpower, physical resources, socio-economic developments, organisation of health care and general health outcomes, illustrated in a comparison between Israel, Canada and Kenya | Ellencweig (1992) |
| | | Seven models described, based on two criteria: type of finance (voluntary or compulsory) and method of paying providers (directly by consumers with or without insurance, indirectly by third parties by contracts, and by budgets and salaries within an integrated organisation) | Hurst (1992) |
| | | Describes a five-category typology for comparing different groups of nations' health systems, based on a theory of the worldwide division of labour combined with the strength of the workers' movement | Elling (1994) |

| Type of study Comparison of | Sub-type Comparison of | Details | Reference |
|---|---|---|---|
| 7 HEALTH CARE REFORMS | | | |
| | OECD countries | Comparison of health reforms in the OECD countries | OECD (1994); Hurst (1992) |
| | Europe | Comparison of reforms in Europe using the WHO information and knowledge base on health care reforms – see also papers for the 1996 Ljubljana conference. In 1996 detailed reports were produced for six countries using a standard description of the system and reforms ('HIT' reports) | WHO (1996b) |
| | Reforms in developing countries | Discussion of methods for improving comparisons of health reforms in developing countries, especially South America, including minimum dataset for comparative reform analysis and a description of the International Clearinghouse for Health System Reform Initiatives to stimulate shred learning | Block (1997) |
| | In-country comparison | Comparison of changes and effects on health indicators of the 1990 reform programme on an urban and a rural area of Zimbabwe | Bijlmakers *et al.* (1996) |
| | Concepts | A conceptual comparison of European health care reform, presenting similarities and differences in aims and actions | Saltman (1994) |
| | Methodology | Methodological problems in comparing health care reforms which also apply to any policy and intervention to organisation comparison. Includes a description of a simple 'Reform Implementation Index' which represents the extent of implementation before and after the formal date, and which allows a statistical analysis of the reform effect | Kroneman & van der Zee (1997) |
| 8 HEALTH AND HEALTH CARE POLICIES | | | |
| | Osteoporosis testing | Compares how bone density measurement has been adopted in different ways in Sweden and Australia and explains this in terms of differences in each country of characteristics of the health care systems, technology assessments, and health authority policies | Marshall *et al.* (1996) |

| Type of study<br>Comparison of | Sub-type<br>Comparison of | Details | Reference |
|---|---|---|---|
| | Different policies for diffusing knowledge | Compares and explains the slow diffusion of understanding of the role of sleeping position in the aetiology of sudden infant death syndrome in the Netherlands, New Zealand, UK and Scandinavia. Short discussion of problems in international policy comparisons: the need to involve many respondents in each country because of differences in recall, the unavailability or delays in outcome data, problems in time series analysis (contamination of adjacent areas, the effects of phased intervention and simultaneous events that affect death rates) | Mckee *et al.* (1996) |
| | Policies to reduce inequalities in health and accessibility | Comparison of the implementation of policy to decrease regional differences in health status and accessibility to health services. Compares data on inequalities from existing sources, and notes the limitations of these sources | Samela (1993); Rosen & Thelle (1996) |
| | Methods for managing the gap between demand and resources | Comparison of approaches to managing the difference between demand and resources for public health care and of approaches to rationing | Øvretveit (1997a) |
| | Patients' rights | Comparison of patients' rights and consumer guarantees in Europe | Fallberg (1996) |
| | Priorities | Comparison of systems for setting priorities and issues in six countries. Publication of papers and discussion for a seminar in UK | Honingsbaum *et al.* (1996) |
| | WHO 'health for all' policy and programme | WHO (1981a) describes indicators to be used to assess progress of the policy 'Health for all by the year 2000'. WHO (1994) reports a comparison by WHO of the progress of different countries from data provided by the countries according to format supplied by WHO | WHO (1981a)<br><br>WHO (1994) |

| Type of study Comparison of | Sub-type Comparison of | Details | Reference |
|---|---|---|---|
| 9 OTHER COMPARISONS | | | |
| | Per capita gross domestic product | Raw statistics | OECD (1993) |
| | Unemployment rate | Raw statistics | Eurostat (1992) |
| | Level of education | Raw statistics | Eurostat (1992) |
| | 'Human development index' | The index combines life expectancy, literacy, and average income. Is used by the United Nations Development Programme | Reference unknown |
| | % of live births | To mothers under 20, 1981–89 | WHO (1992) |
| | Comparability of different economic evaluations undertaken in different countries | The same economic evaluation of a drug was undertaken in four countries using the same methods. This study considers whether a standard method could be agreed in different countries to ensure comparability of findings and to compare differences in costs and benefits in different countries | Drummond *et al.* (1992) |

# Further reading

Appleby J, Smith P, Ranade W *et al.* (1994) Monitoring managed competition. In: *Evaluating the NHS Reforms* (eds R Robinson and J Le Grand), pp. 24–35. Kings Fund Institute, London.

Appleby J, Walshe K and Ham C (1995) *Acting on the Evidence: a review of clinical effectiveness – sources of information, dissemination and implementation.* NAHAT, Birmingham.

Bardsley M and Coles J (1992) Practical experiences in auditing patient outcomes. *Quality in Health Care* 1: 124–30.

Berger PL and Luckman T (1967) *The Social Construction of Reality.* Allen Lane, London.

Brooks T (1992) Success through organisational audit. *Health Services Management.* Nov/Dec: 13–15.

Brooks T and Pitt C (1990) The standard bearers. *Health Services Journal.* 30 August: 1286–7.

Buck N, Devlin H, Lunn J (1987) *Report of a confidential enquiry into perioperative deaths.* Nuffield Provincial Hospitals Trust, London.

CEPPP (1991) *Evaluation of TQM in the NHS: first interim report.* CEPPP, Brunel University.

Cochrane A (1972) *Effectiveness and Efficiency.* Nuffield Provincial Hospitals Trust, London.

DesHarnais S, Laurence F, McMahon Jnr and Wroblewski R (1991) Measuring outcomes of hospital care using risk-adjusted indexes. *Health Services Research* 26: 425–45.

Dixon P and Carr-Hill R (1989) *The NHS and its Customers III: consumer feedback – A review of current practice.* Centre of Health Economics, University of York.

DoH (1989) *Report on confidential enquiries into maternal deaths in England and Wales 1982–84.* HMSO, London.

Donabedian A (1980) *Exploration in Quality Assessment and Monitoring Volume I. Definition of Quality and Approaches to its Assessment.* Health Administration Press, University of Michigan, Ann Arbor.

Drummond M (1987) *Economic Appraisal of Health Technology in the European Community.* Oxford University Press, Oxford.

Drummond M (1987) Economic evaluation and the rational diffusion and use of health technology. *Health Policy* 7: 309–24.

Edgren L (1995) *Evaluation of the SPRI Version of Organisational Audit at Lund University Hospital.* The Nordic School of Public Health, Goteborg. (Summary in English.)

EFQM (1992) *The European Quality Award 1992.* European Foundation for Quality Management, Brussels, Belgium.

Ellis R and Whittington D (1993) *Quality Assurance in Health Care: A handbook.* Edward Arnold, London.

Flanagan J (1954) The Critical Incident Technique. *Psychological Bulletin* 5: 327–58.

Fowkes F and Fulton P (1991) Critical appraisal of published research: introductory guidelines. *BMJ* 302: 1136–40.

Gerard K and Mooney G (1993) QALY league tables: handle with care. *Health Economics* 2: 59–64.

Giddens A (1974) *Positivism and Sociology.* Heinemann, London.

Glaser BG and Strauss AL (1968) *The Discovery of Grounded Theory: strategies for qualitative research.* Weidenfeld & Nicolson, London.

Ham C and Woolley M (1996) *How does the NHS measure up? Assessing the performance of health authorities.* National Association of Health Authorities and Trusts, Birmingham.

Harper J (1986) Measuring performance – a new approach. *Hospital and Health Services Review.* Jan: 26–8.

Harrison S, Hunter D and Pollitt C (1990) *The Dynamics of British Health Policy.* Unwin Hyman, London.

Helman C (1994) *Culture, Health and Illness.* Butterworth Heinemann, London.

Johnston N, Narayan V and Ruta D (1992) Development of indicators for quality assurance in public health medicine. *Quality in Health Care* **1**: 225–30.

Jones R (1995) Why do qualitative research? *BMJ* **311**: 2.

Joss R, Kogan M and Henkel M (1994) *Final Report to the Department of Health on Total Quality Management Experiments in the National Health Service.* Centre for Evaluation of Public Policy and Practice, Brunel University, Middlesex.

Keesing R (1981) *Cultural Anthropology: a contemporary perspective.* Holt, Rienhart & Winston, New York.

Kerrison S, Packwood T and Buxton M (1993) *Medical Audit: taking stock.* Kings Fund, London.

Klein R and Scrivens E (1993) The bottom line – accreditation in the UK. *Health Services Journal.* 25 November: 25–6.

Kogan M and Redfern S (eds) (1995) *Making Use of Clinical Audit: a guide to practice in the health professions.* Open University Press, Milton Keynes.

Leech E (1982) *Social Anthropology.* Fontana, Glasgow.

Long A, Dixon P, Hall R *et al.* (1993) The outcomes agenda. *Quality In Health Care* **2**: 49–52.

Lonner W and Berry J (eds) (1986) *Field Methods in Cross-Cultural Research.* Sage, London.

Mahaparatra P and Berman P (1994) Using hospital activity indicators to evaluate performance in Andra Pradesh, India. *International Journal of Health Planning and Management* **9**: 199–211.

Majeed F and Voss S (1995) Performance indicators for general practice. *BMJ* **311**: 209–10.

Marmot M *et al.* (1975) *American Journal of Epidemiology* **102**: 514–25.

Mays N and Pope C (1995) Rigour and qualitative research. *BMJ* **311**: 109–13.

Miller P (1997) Are GP fundholders wasting money? *Health Services Journal.* 6 March: 28–9.

NIST (1990) *The Malcum Baldridge National Quality Award 1990 Application Guidelines.* National Institute of Standards and Technology, Gaithersburg, MD 20899, USA.

Nordberg E, Oganga H, Kazibwe S and Onyango J (1993) Rapid assessment of an African district health system. *International Journal of Health Planning and Management* **8**: 219–33.

OECD (1995) *Health Data File, version 3.6.* Organisation for Economic Co-operation and Development, Paris.

Øyen E (ed) (1990) *Comparative Methodology.* Sage, London.

PHCCCC (1992) *Hospital Effectiveness Report.* Pennsylvania Health Care Cost Containment Council, Harrison Transport Centre, Suite 2-F, Harrisburg, PA 17101.

Pollitt C (1992) *The Politics of Medical Quality: auditing doctors in the UK and the USA.* Unpublished draft, Dept. of Government, Brunel University, Uxbridge, Middlesex.

Pope C and Mays N (1995) Reaching the parts other methods cannot reach: an introduction to qualitative methods in health and health services research. *BMJ* **311**: 42–5.

Rhodes G, Wiley M, Tomas J *et al.* (1997) Comparing EU hospital efficiency using DRGs. *European Journal of Public Health* **7** (3): 42–50.

Roberts H (1990) *Outcome and Performance in Health Care.* Public Finance Foundation, London.

Robinson R and Le Grand J (1994) *Evaluating the NHS Reforms.* Kings Fund Institute, London.

Rose R (1991) Comparing forms of comparative analysis. *Political Studies* **39**: 446–62.

Saltman R and Figuras J (eds) (1997) *European Health Care Reform: analysis of current strategies.* WHO, Copenhagen (European Series No. 72).

Schelesselman J (1982) *Case–Control Studies: design, conduct, analysis.* Oxford University Press, Oxford.

Schwartz D, Flamant R and Lellouch J (1980) *Clinical Trials.* Academic Press, London.

Schyve P (1995) Models for relating performance measurement and accreditation. *International Journal of Health Planning and Management* **10**: 231–41.

Scott A and Hall J (1995) Evaluating the effects of GP remuneration: problems and prospects. *Health Policy and Planning* **31**: 183–95.

Strauss A and Corbin J (1990) *Basics of Qualitative Research.* Sage, London.

Usherwood T (1996) *Introduction to Project Management in Health Research: a guide for new researchers.* Open University Press, Milton Keynes.

Walshe K and Coles J (1993) *Evaluating Audit: a review of initiatives.* CASPE Research, London.

Walt G (1994) *Health Policy: an introduction to process and power.* Zed Books, London.

Webb E, Campell D, Schwarz R and Sechrest L (1966) *Unobtrusive measures: nonreactive research in the social sciences.* Rand McNally, Chicago.

WHO (1981) *Health Programme Evaluation.* World Health Organisation, Geneva.

WHO (1994) *Evaluation of Recent Changes in the Financing of Health Services.* World Health Organisation, Geneva.

Øvretveit J (1984) *Is Action Research Scientific? – Social analysis and action research.* Unpublished Master Thesis, Brunel University, Uxbridge.

Øvretveit J (1993) *Coordinating Community Care: multidisciplinary teams and care management in health and social services.* Open University Press, Milton Keynes.

Øvretveit J (1993) *Measuring Service Quality.* Technical Communications Publications Ltd., Aylesbury, Herts.

Øvretveit J (1994) *Purchasing for Health.* Open University Press, Milton Keynes.

Øvretveit J (1996) *Health Evaluation – a learning resource pack for public health programmes.* The Nordic School of Public Health, Goteborg.

Øvretveit J (1997a) Learning from quality improvement in Europe and beyond. *Journal of the Joint Commission for Accreditation of Healthcare Organisations* **23**: 7–22.

Øvretveit J (1997b) A comparison of hospital quality programmes – lessons for other services. *International Journal of Service Industry Management* **8**: 220–35.

# References

Adams G and Shvaneveldt J (1991) *Understanding Research Methods.* Longman, New York.

Alban A and Christiansen T (eds) (1995) *The Nordic Lights: new initiatives in health care systems.* Odense University Press, Odense.

Appleby J (1993) Health and efficiency. *Health Services Journal.* 6 May: 20–2.

Appleby J (1996) Promoting efficiency in the NHS: problems with the labour productivity index. *BMJ* **313**: 1319–21.

Armatage P and Berry G (1987) *Statistical Methods in Medical Research.* Blackwell, Oxford.

Bijlmakers L, Basset M and Sanders D (1996) *Health and Structural Adjustment in Rural and Urban Zimbabwe.* The Scandinavian Institute of African Studies, Research report No. 101, Uppsala.

Black T (1993) *Evaluating Social Science Research.* Sage, London.

Block M (1997) Comparative research and analysis methods for shared learning from health system reforms. *Health Policy* **42**: 187–209.

Boshuizen H, van de Water H and Penenboom R (1994) *International comparison of health expectancy.* TNO Prevention and Health, Leiden, the Netherlands.

Bowling A (1992) *Measuring Health: a review of quality of life measures.* Open University Press, Milton Keynes.

Bowling A (1995) *Measuring Disease: a reveiw of disease-specific quality of life measurement scales.* Open University Press, Milton Keynes.

Boys R, Forster D and Jozan P (1991) Mortality from causes amenable and non-amenable to medical care: the experience of Eastern Europe. *BMJ* **303**: 879–83.

Bradshaw J (1972) A taxonomy of social need. In: *Problems and Progress in Medical Care* (ed G McLachlan). Oxford University Press, London.

Breakwell G and Millward L (1995) *Basic Evaluation Methods*. British Psychological Society Books, Leicester.

Britten, N (1995) Qualitative interviews in medical research. *BMJ* **311**: 251–3.

Buchan J (1997) The states we're in. *Health Services Journal*. 24 April: 27–9.

Campbell H, Hotchkiss R, Bradshaw N and Porteous J (1998) Integrated care pathways. *BMJ* **316**: 133–7.

CEC (1988) *Europeans and cancer prevention: a study of attitudes and behaviour of the public.* Commission of the European Communities, DG for Employment, Brussels.

CEC (1991) *Prevention of women's cancers: cancers of the cervix and breast – early diagnosis and screening.* Commission of the European Communities, Brussels.

Chassin M, Brook R, Part R *et al.* (1986) Variations in the use of medical and surgical services by the Medicare population. *New England Journal of Medicine* **314**: 285–9.

Cook T and Campbell D (1979) *Quasi-experimentation: design and analysis issues in field settings.* Rand McNally, Chicago.

Crombie I (1996) *The Pocket Guide to Critical Appraisal.* British Medical Journal, London.

Denzin N and Lincoln Y (eds) (1993) *Handbook of Qualitative Research.* Sage, London.

Domenighetti G, Luraschi P, Gutzwiller F *et al.* (1988) Effect of information changes by the mass media on hysterectomy rates. *Lancet* **2**: 1470-3.

Doorslaer E, Wagstaff A and Rutten F (eds) (1994) *Equity in the Finance and Delivery of Health Care. An International Perspective.* Oxford University Press, Oxford.

Drummond M, Bloom B, Carrin G *et al.* (1992) Issues in the cross-national assessment of health technology. *International Journal of Technology Assessment in Health Care* **8**: 671–82.

Drummond M, Stoddard G and Torrence G (1987) *Methods for the Economic Evaluation of Health Care Programmes.* Oxford Medical Publications, Oxford.

Edwards A and Talbot R (1994) *The Hard-Pressed Researcher.* Longman, London.

Ellencweig A (1992) *Analysing Health Systems. A modular approach*. Oxford University Press, Oxford.

Elling R (1994) Theory and method for the cross-national study of health systems. *International Journal of Health Services* **24**: 285–309.

Eurostat (1992) *Facts Through Figures*. Office for Official Publications of the European Communities, Luxembourg.

Evstifeeva T, MacFarlanne G and Robertson C (1997) Trends in cancer mortality in central European countries. *European Journal of Public Health* **7**: 169–76.

Fallberg L (1996) Patients' rights. In: *Citizen Choice and Patients' Rights in European Health Reform*. WHO, Copenhagen.

Fink A (1993) *Evaluation Fundamentals*. Sage, London.

Fink J, Jensen J, Borgquist L *et al*. (1995) Psychiatric morbidity in primary health care. A Nordic multicentre investigation. Part 1. Methods and prevalence of psychiatric morbidity. *Acta Psychiatrica Scandinavia* **92**: 409–18.

Fitzpatrick R and Boulton M (1994) Qualitative methods for assessing health care. *Quality in Health Care* **3**: 107–13.

Fletcher C, Jones N, Burrows B and Niden A (1994) American emphysema and British bronchitis: a standardized comparative study. *American Review of Respiratory Diseases* **90**: 1–13.

Frankfort-Nachmias C and Nachmias D (1992) *Research Methods in Social Sciences* (4th edn). Edward Arnold, London.

Frohlich N and Mustard C (1996) A regional comparison of socio-economic and health indices in a Canadian province. *Social Science and Medicine* **42**: 1273–81.

Gardner M and Altman D (1989) *Statistics with Confidence*. British Medical Journal, London.

Garpenby P and Carlsson P (1994) The role of national quality registers in the Swedish health service. *Health Policy* **29**: 183–95.

Ghauri P, Grønhaug K and Kristianslund I (1995) *Research Methods in Business Studies*. Prentice Hall, London.

Gissler M, Teperi J, Hemminki E and Merilainen J (1995) Data quality after restructuring a National Medical Registry. *Scandinavian Journal of Social Medicine* **23**: 75–80.

Golden B (1992) The past is the past – or is it? The use of retrospective accounts as indicators of past strategy. *Academy of Management Journal* **35**: 848–60.

Gray M (1997) *Evidence-based healthcare*. Churchill Livingstone, London.

Grimshaw J, Freemantle N, Wallace S *et al.* (1995) Developing and implementing clinical practice guidelines. *Quality in Health Care* **4**: 55-64.

Guldvog B, Hofoss G, Ebbesen J and Pettersen K (1995) *RESQUA: A program for outcomes research and quality improvement in hospitals*. Foundation for Health Services Research (HELTEF), PB 55, N-1474, Nordbyhagen, Norway.

Ham C (ed) (1997) *Health Care Reform*. Open University Press, Milton Keynes.

Ham C, Robinson R and Benzeval M (1990) *Health Check: health care reforms in an international context*. Kings Fund, London.

Helzer J and Canino G (eds) (1992) *Alcoholism in North America, Europe and Asia*. Oxford University Press, Oxford.

Holland W (ed) (1983) *Evaluation of Health Care*. Oxford University Press, Oxford.

Honigsbaum F, Holmstrom S and Calltorp J (1996) *Making Choices in Health Care*. Radcliffe Medical Press, Oxford.

Hopton J and Dlugolecka M (1995) Need and demand for primary health care: a comparative survey approach. *BMJ* **310**: 1369–73.

Hurst J (1992) The reform of health care: a comparative analysis of seven OECD countries. Health Policy Studies No. 2, Organisation for Economic Co-operation and Development, Paris.

IHSM (1990) *Models of Clinical Management*. Institute of Health Service Management, London.

Jarman B (1983) Indentification of underprivileged areas. *BMJ* **286**: 1705.

Jick T (1983) Mixing qualitative and quantitative methods: triangulation in action. In: *Qualitative Methodology* (ed J Van Maanen). Sage, Beverly Hills.

Johansson L *et al.* (1997) Suicide among foreign-born minorities and native Swedes: an epidemiological follow-up study of a defined population. *Social Science and Medicine* **44**: 181–7.

Joss R and Kogan M (1995) *Advancing Quality*. Open University Press, Milton Keynes.

Kelly G (1955) *A Theory of Personality.* Norton, New York.

Kerlinger F (1986) *Foundations of Behavioral Research.* Holt, Rinehart & Winston, New York.

Kessler R, Frank R, Edlund M *et al.* (1997) Differences in the use of psychiatric outpatient services between the USA and Ontario. *New England Journal of Medicine* **336**: 551–7.

Kitzinger J (1995) Introducing focus groups. *BMJ* **311**: 299–302.

Kreuger R (1988) *Focus Groups: a practical guide for applied research.* Sage, London.

Kristiansen I and Mooney G (1993) Remuneration of GP services. *Health Policy* **24**: 203–12.

Kroneman M and van der Zee J (1997) Health policy as a fuzzy concept: methodological problems encountered when evaluating health policy reforms in an international perspective. *Health Policy* **40**: 139–55.

Kvale S (1989) *Issues of Validity in Qualitative Research.* Studentlitteratur, Lund.

Kvale S (1994) Ten standard objections to qualitative research interviews. *Journal of Phenomenological Psychology*: 1–28.

Leape L, Edward Park R, Soloman D *et al.* (1990) Does inappropriate use explain small-area variations in the use of health services. *Journal of the American Medical Association* **263**: 669–72.

Lewinter M (1997) *A comparison of Danish and Swedish Services for Older People.* Nordic School of Public Health, Goteborg.

Leyland A and Boddy A (1997) Measuring performance in hospital care: length of stay in Gynaecology. *European Journal of Public Health* **7**: 136–43.

Madsen M (1996) Nordic variations in surgical operation rates. In: *Sygehusvaesenet mod år 2000* (ed F Kamper-Jørgensen). Dike, Copenhagen.

Marmot M and Syme S (1976) Acculturation and coronary heart disease in Japanese Americans. *American Journal of Epidemiology* **104**: 225–47.

Marshall D, Hailey D and Jonsson E (1996) Health policy on bone density measurement technology in Sweden and Australia. *Health Policy* **35**: 217–28.

Mays N and Pope C (1995) Observational methods in health care settings. *BMJ* **311**: 182–4.

McConway K (ed) (1994) *Studying Health and Disease.* Open University Press, Milton Keynes.

Mckee M *et al.* (1996) Preventing sudden infant deaths: the slow diffusion of an idea. *Health Policy* **37**: 117–35.

Mckee M and Hunter D (1995) Mortality league tables: do they inform or mislead? *Quality in Health Care* **4**: 5–12.

McKinlay J (1992) Advantages and limitations of the survey approach – understanding older people. In: *Researching Health Care: designs, dilemmas, disciplines* (eds J Daly, I McDonald and E Willis), pp. 114–37. Routledge, London.

McPherson K (1989) International differences in medical care practices. *Health Care Financing Review, Annual Supplement*: 9–20.

McPherson K, Wennberg J, Hovind O and Clifford P (1982) Small area variation in the use of common surgical procedures: an international comparison in New England, England and Norway. *New England Journal of Medicine* **307**: 1310–14.

Middle C and Macfarlane A (1995) Recorded delivery. *Health Service Journal.* 31 Aug: 27.

Miles M and Huberman A (1984) *Qualitative Data Analysis: a source book of new methods.* Sage, Beverly Hills, California.

Morgan D (ed) (1993) *Successful Focus Groups.* Sage, London.

Mossialos E (1997) Citizens' views on health systems in the 15 member states of the European Union. *Health Economics* **6**: 109–16.

Munk-Jørgensen P, Fink J and Brevik J (1997) Psychiatric morbidity in primary health care: a multicentre investigation. Part II. Hidden morbidity and choice of treatment. *Acta Psychiatrica Scandinavia* **95**: 6–12.

Najman J, Morrison J, Williams G and Anderson M (1992) Comparing alternative methodologies of social research. In: *Researching Health Care: designs, dilemmas, disciplines* (eds J Daly, I McDonald and E Willis), pp. 114–37. Routledge, London.

Nathanson C (1978) Sex roles as a variable in the interpretation of morbidity data: a methodological critique. *International Journal of Epidemiology* **7**: 253–62. (From the Danish National Morbidity Survey)

NCEPOD (1987, 1989) *Report of a National Confidential Enquiry into Perioperative Deaths.* Kings Fund, London.

NCEPOD (1993) *Report of the National Confidential Enquiry into Perioperative Deaths, 1991/92.* 35 Lincoln's Inn Fields, London WC2 3PN.

NCM (1995) *Yearbook of Nordic Statistics 1995.* Nordic Council of Ministers, Copenhagen.

NHSCR&D (1996) *Undertaking systematic reviews of research on effectiveness: CRD guidelines for carrying out or commissioning reviews.* NHS Centre for Reviews and Dissemination, York University.

Nilssen O, Lipton R, Brenn T *et al.* (1997) Sleeping problems at 78 degrees north: the Svalbard study. *Acta Psychiatrica Scandinavia* **95**: 44–8.

NOMESCO (1996) *Health Statistics in the Nordic Countries 1994.* Nordic Medico Statistical Committee, Copenhagen.

O'Brien B (1984) *Patterns of European Diagnosis and Prescribing.* Office of Health Economics, London.

OECD (1987) *Financing and Delivering Health Care, a comparative analysis of OECD countries.* Organisation for Economic Co-operation and Development, Paris.

OECD (1990) *Health Care Systems in Transition: the search for efficiency (Compendium: health care expenditure and other data).* Policy Studies No 7, Organisation for Economic Co-operation and Development, Paris.

OECD (1992) *The Reform of Healthcare Systems: a comparative analysis of seven OECD countries.* Organisation for Economic Co-operation and Development, Paris.

OECD (1993a) *OECD Health Data: comparative analysis of health systems.* Organisation for Economic Co-operation and Development, Paris.

OECD (1993b) *OECD Health Systems, Facts and Trends 1960–1991.* Organisation for Economic Co-operation and Development, Paris.

OECD (1994) *The Reform of Healthcare Systems: a review of seventeen OECD countries.* Organisation for Economic Co-operation and Development, Paris.

Ong B (1993) *The Practice of Health Service Research.* Chapman & Hall, London.

Ong B, Humpris G, Annett H and Rafkin S (1991) Rapid appraisal in an urban setting – an example from the developed world. *Social Science and Medicine* **32**: 9015.

OU (1973) *Methods of Educational Enquiry, E 341. Block 2: Research design,* pp. 19–21. Open University Press, Milton Keynes.

Packwood T, Keen J and Buxton M (1991) *Hospitals in Transition: The resource management experiment.* Open University Press, Milton Keynes.

Patton M (1987) *How to Use Qualitative Methods in Evaluation*. Sage, London.

Pettigrew A, Ferlie E and McKee L (1992) *Shaping Strategic Change*. Sage, London.

Phillips C, Palfry C and Thomas P (1994) *Evaluating Health and Social Care*. Macmillan, London.

Pocock S (1983) *Clinical Trials: a practical approach*. John Wiley, Chichester.

Powell J, Lovelock R, Bray J and Philp I (1994) Involving consumers in assessing service quality using a qualitative approach. *Quality in Health Care* 3: 199–202.

Poullier J (1989) Health care expenditure and other data. *Health Care Financing Review* (annual supplement): 111–18.

RCGP (1992) *The European Study of Referrals from Primary to Secondary Care*. Royal College of General Practitioners, London.

Rehnberg C (1997) Sweden. In: *Health Care Reform* (ed C Ham). Open University Press, Milton Keynes.

Reif K and Ingelhart R (1991) *Eurobarometer: the dynamics of public opinion*. Macmillan, London.

Rosen M (1987) *Epidemiology in Planning for Health*. Department of Social Medicine, Umeå.

Rosen M and Thelle D (1996) *Cardiovascular Diseases in the Nordic Countries*. NOMESCO, Copenhagen.

Rossi P and Freeman H (1993) *Evaluation – a systematic approach*. Sage, London.

Sackett D, Rosenberg W, Gray J, Haynes R and Scott-Richardson W (1996) Evidence-based medicine: what it is and what it isn't. *BMJ* **312**: 71–2.

Saltman R (1994) A conceptual overview of recent health care reforms. *European Journal of Public Health* **4**: 287–93.

Saltman R and Figuras J (eds) (1998) *Critical Challenges for Healthcare Reform in Europe*. Milton Keynes, Open University Press.

Samela R (1993) Regional inequalities in health and health care in Finland and Norway. *Health Policy* **24**: 83–94.

Sapsford R and Abbott P (1992) *Research Methods for Nurses and the Caring Professions*. Open University Press, Milton Keynes.

Schaapveld K, Chorus A and Perenboom R (1995) The European health potential: what can we learn from each other. *Health Policy* **33**: 205–17.

Scrivens E (1995) *Accreditation: protecting the professional or the consumer.* Open University Press, Milton Keynes.

Shieber G and Poullier J (1989) Overview of international comparisons of healthcare expenditure. *Health Care Financing Review* (annual supplement): 111–18.

Sketris I (1988) *Health Service Accreditation – an international overview.* Kings Fund Centre, London.

Slevin C and Stuart A (1978) Data dredging procedures in survey analysis. In: *Social Research: Principles and Procedures* (eds J Bynner and K Stvibly), pp. 278–84. Longman, London.

Smith M, Glass G and Miller T (1980) *The Benefits of Psychotherapy.* Johns Hopkins University Press, Baltimore, MD.

Stano M (1993) Evaluating the policy role of the small area variation and physician practice style hypothesis. *Health Policy* **24**: 9–17.

Stiles T *et al.* (1993) WHO (Nordic) multicentre study on parasuicide. *Nordic Journal of Psychiatry* **47**: 281–6.

St Leger A, Schienden H and Walsworth-Bell J (1992) *Evaluating Health Service Effectiveness.* Open Univeristy Press, Milton Keynes.

Sundquist J and Johansson S (1997) Long-term illness among indigenous and foreign-born people in Sweden. *Social Science and Medicine* **44**: 189–98.

Thompson R, McElroy H and Kazandjian V (1997) Maryland hospital quality indicator project in the UK. *Quality in Health Care* **6**: 49–55.

Townsend P, Phillimore P and Beattie J (1988) *Health and Deprivation. Inequality and the North.* Croom Helm, London.

Vallgårda S (1996) Hospitalisation of deliveries: the change of place of birth in Denmark and Sweden from the late nineteenth century to 1970. *Medical History* **40**: 173–96.

van de Vijver F and Leung K (1997) *Methods and Data Analysis for Cross-cultural Research.* Sage, London.

van de Water H, Perenboom R and Boshuizen H (1996) Policy relevance of the health expectancy indicator: an inventory in European Union countries. *Health Policy* **36**: 117–29.

Van Maanen J (ed) (1983) *Qualitative Methodology.* Sage, Beverly Hills, CA.

Van Os J, Galdos P, Lewis G *et al.* (1993) Schizophrenia san frontieres: concepts of schizophrenia among French and British psychiatrists. *BMJ* **307**: 489–92.

Vlassoff C and Tanner M (1992) The relevance of rapid assessment to health research and interventions. *Health Policy and Planning* **7**: 1–9.

Walshe K (1997) Indicators won't turn the tables. *Health Services Journal*. 17 July: 24.

WHO (1981) *Development of Indicators for Monitoring Progress Towards Health for All by the Year 2000*. World Health Organisation, Geneva.

WHO (1992) *Eurostat (HFA Indicators) Programme*. WHO-Euro, Copenhagen.

WHO (1994) *Implementation of the Global Strategy for Health For All by the Year 2000 – second evaluation. Eighth report of the world health situation*. World Health Organisation, Geneva. (Note: volume 5 is the European Region Report. First evaluation was in 1988)

WHO (1996a) *The Health of Youth: a cross-national survey*. World Health Organisation, Copenhagen.

WHO (1996b) *Health Care Reforms in Europe*. World Health Organisation, Copenhagen.

WHO (1997) *Health For All Database*. World Health Organisation, Copenhagen.

Wiley M (1992) Hospital financing reform and case-mix measurement: an international review. *Health Care Financing Review* **13**: 119–33.

Wiltkin D, Hallan L and Dogget M (1992) *Measures of Need and Outcome for Primary Health Care*. Oxford Medical Publications, Oxford.

Woolhandler S and Himmelstein D (1997) Costs of care and administration at for-profit and other hospitals in the United States. *New England Journal of Medicine* **336**: 769–74.

World Bank (1993) *World Development Report 1993 – investing in health*. Oxford University Press, New York.

Yin R (1981) The case study crisis: some answers. *Administrative Science Quarterly* **26**: 58–65.

Yin R (1994) *Case Study Research: design and methods*. Sage, Beverly Hills, CA.

Øvretveit J (1988) *A Peer Review Process for Developing Service Quality.* BIOSS Working Paper, Brunel University, Uxbridge, Middlesex.

Øvretveit J (1991) *Primary Care Quality Through Teamwork.* Research Report, BIOSS, Brunel University, Uxbridge, Middlesex.

Øvretveit J (1992) *Health Service Quality.* Blackwell Scientific, Oxford.

Øvretveit J (1994a) Values in European Health Care Reforms. *European Journal of Public Health* 4(2): 26–36.

Øvretveit J (1994b) A comparison of approaches to quality in the UK, USA and Sweden, and of the use of organisational audit frameworks. *European Journal of Public Health* 4(1): 46–54.

Øvretveit J (1994c) A framework for cost-effective team quality and multi-professional audit. *Journal of Interprofessional Care* 8: 329–33.

Øvretveit J (1996a) Informed choice? Patient access to health service quality information. *Health Policy* 36: 75–93.

Øvretveit J (1996b) *The Quality Journeys of Five Norwegian Hospitals.* Norwegian Medical Association, Lysaker, Norway.

Øvretveit J (1997a) Managing the gaps between demand and publically-affordable health care. *European Journal of Public Health* 7: 128–35.

Øvretveit J (1997b) *Cooperation in Mental Health Services in Three Scandinavian Areas.* The Nordic School of Public Health, Goteborg, Sweden.

Øvretveit, J (1997c) Evidence-based management technologies. *Journal of Health Gain.* Autumn: 1–5.

Øvretveit J (1998) *Evaluating Health Interventions.* Open University Press, Milton Keynes.

Øvretveit J and Aslaksen A (1997) *Evaluation of the Norwegian Total Quality Programme – second report.* Norwegian Medical Association, Lysaker, Norway.

Øvretveit J and Aslaksen A (1998) The Quality Journeys of Six Norwegian hospitals: final report of an evaluation of the Norwegian Total Quality Management Programme. Norwegian Medical Association, Oslo, Norway.

# Index